Rapid
Surgery

RAPID
SURGERY

Ebube E. Obi

Cara R. Baker

James T.H. Teo
All of Royal Free and University College Medical School
University College London
London

Mark T.W. Teo
University of Nottingham Medical School
Nottingham

EDITORIAL ADVISOR
Brian Davidson
Professor of Surgery
Royal Free and University College Medical School
University College London
London

SERIES EDITOR
Amir H. Sam
Royal Free and University College Medical School
University College London
London

Blackwell
Publishing

© 2005 by Blackwell Publishing Ltd
Published by Blackwell Publishing Ltd
Blackwell Publishing, Inc., 350 Main Street, Malden,
  Massachusetts 02148-5020, USA
Blackwell Publishing Ltd, 9600 Garsington Road, Oxford OX4 2DQ, UK
Blackwell Publishing Asia Pty Ltd, 550 Swanston Street, Carlton,
  Victoria 3053, Australia

First published 2005

Library of Congress Cataloging-in-Publication Data

Rapid surgery / Ebube E. Obi ... [et al.] ; editorial advisor, Brian
Davidson.
     p. ; cm. – (Rapid series)
   Includes bibliographical references.
   ISBN 1-4051-1435-0
1. Surgery–Handbooks, manuals, etc.
   [DNLM: 1. Surgery–Handbooks. WO 39 R218 2005] I. Obi, Ebube E.
II. Series.

   RD37.R375 2005
   617–dc22   2004009508

ISBN-13: 978-1-4051-1435-6
ISBN-10: 1-4051-1435-5

A catalogue record for this title is available from the British Library

Set in Frutiger 7/9pt by Kolam Information Services Pvt. Ltd,
Pondicherry, India
Printed and bound in India by Replika Press Pvt. Ltd

Commissioning Editor: Vicki Noyes
Editorial Assistant: Nicola Ulyatt
Production Editor: Lorna Hind
Production Controller: Kate Charman

For further information on Blackwell Publishing, visit our website:
http://www.blackwellpublishing.com

All the medical illustrations are provided by Ebube Obi.

CONTENTS

Specialties

CONTENTS

Procedures

CONTENTS

In the conception of this book, we envisaged a text presented in a very accessible format covering the major surgical specialties. We have included surgical procedures – something that is lacking in most textbooks. Also included are radiographs of numerous conditions to aid in consolidating learning. The drawings help to visualise difficult concepts, e.g. suturing, amputations.

This book describes 113 common surgical conditions, 33 practical surgical procedures, and has over 30 illustrations. Sections describing surgical conditions have been subdivided into 11 structured subheadings based on the Rapid Series Mnemonic in list 1. The surgical procedures follow the six subheadings in list 2. We hope that this textbook will consolidate your personal and ward-based learning and that you will enjoy reading it.

This work would not have been possible without the invaluable unwavering support and assistance of Professor Brian Davidson MD, FRCS. We would like to thank our consultants at the Royal Free Hospital for their advice and help in reviewing our work: Miss C. Davey, FRCOPhth; Mr T. Davidson, ChM MRCP FRCS; Mr N. Garlick, FRCS (Orth); Dr J. Hinton, MRCP, FRCR; Mr C. Shieff, MBChB FRCS.

We would also like to thank the Department of Radiology for granting us access to use the radiographs of the Royal Free Hospital Radiology Library. Finally, we would like to acknowledge those who have been an inspiration to us at the Royal Free Hospital, especially Mr J. Kirk and Mr J. Norton.

Ebube Obi
Cara Baker
James Teo
Mark Teo

In business 'the customer is always correct'. With a text book on surgery aimed at final year medical students and junior doctors, who better to dictate the format and produce the text than a group of recently qualified medical students? The task of providing the optimal surgical revision text has been taken as a challenge to this accomplished group and has resulted in an invaluable guide through surgical practice. This is a no-frills text book which provides comprehensive coverage of the essentials of general surgical practice, including the diagnosis, investigation and treatment of the conditions commonly encountered. It has the additional advantage of covering the surgical specialities such as orthopaedics, urology and neurosurgery. The information is displayed in a clear and standardised format which allows for easy recollection of facts and these are complemented by a selection of typical illustrations from the radiology archives. I would recommend this text to clinical medical students who want an accurate and comprehensive quick fix guide for surgical revision. However, it would be equally appropriate as a rapid reference guide for junior doctors in at the deep end of surgical practice or other healthcare professionals.

Brian Davidson
September 2004

AAA	abdominal aortic aneurysm		**CVA**	cerebrovascular accident
ABC	airway, breathing, circulation		**CVP**	central venous pressure
ABG	arterial blood gas		**CXR**	chest X-ray
ABPI	ankle–brachial pressure index		**DM**	diabetes mellitus
			DMSA	dimercaptosuccinic acid
ACAG	acute closed-angle glaucoma		**DNA**	deoxyribonucleic acid
ACE	angiotensin-converting enzyme		**DTPA**	diethylenetriamine pentaacetic acid
ACTH	adrenocorticotropic hormone		**DVT**	deep vein thrombosis
			EBV	Epstein–Barr virus
AKA	above-knee amputation		**ECG**	electrocardiogram
			ECST	European Carotid Surgery Trial
AMI	acute myocardial infarction		**EEG**	electroencephalo-gram/graphy
ANDI	aberrations of normal development and involution		**ERCP**	endoscopic retrograde cholangiopancreato-graphy
AP	anteroposterior		**EVAR**	endovascular aortic aneurysm repair
ARDS	acute respiratory distress syndrome		**FAP**	familial adenomatous polyposis
ASA	American Society of Anesthesiologists		**FBC**	full blood count
5-ASA	5-aminosalicylic acid		**FEV**	forced expiratory volume
ATLS	advanced trauma life support		**FFP**	fresh frozen plasma
AV	arteriovenous		**FNA**	fine-needle aspiration
AVM	arteriovenous malformation		**FNAC**	fine-needle aspiration cytology
AXR	abdominal X-ray		**G&S**	group and save
BCG	bacillus Calmette–Guérin		**GCS**	Glasgow Coma Scale
BP	blood pressure		**GI**	gastrointestinal
BPH	benign prostatic hyperplasia		**GIST**	gastrointestinal stromal tumour
CABG	coronary artery bypass grafting		**GORD**	gastro-oesophageal reflux disease
CAVATAS	Carotid and Vertebral Artery Transluminal Angioplasty Study		**HCC**	hepatocellular carcinoma
CEA	carcinoembryonic antigen		**HCG**	human chorionic gonadotropin
			HDU	high dependency unit
CMV	cytomegalovirus		**HIV**	human immunodeficiency virus
CREST	Carotid Revascularization Endarterectomy vs. Stent Trial		**HNPCC**	hereditary nonpolyposis colorectal cancer
CRP	C-reactive protein		**IBD**	inflammatory bowel disease
CSDH	chronic subdural haematoma		**IC**	inspiratory capacity
CT	computed tomography		**ICP**	intracranial pressure

TED	thrombo-embolic deterrent	**TURP**	trans-urethral resection of prostate
TIA	transient ischaemic attack	**U&E**	urea and electrolyte
TNM	tumour, node, metastasis	**UICC**	International Union Against Cancer
tPA	tissue-plasminogen activator	**UMN**	upper motor neuron
TRUS	transrectal ultrasonography	**URTI**	upper respiratory tract infection
TURBT	trans-urethral resection of bladder tumour	**USG**	ultrasonography
		USS	ultrasound scan
		UTI	urinary tract infection
		UV	ultraviolet
		WCC	white cell count

LIST OF ABBREVIATIONS

Rapid series mnemonic

Conditions

D:	Definition	Doctors
A:	Aetiology	Are
A/R:	Associations/Risk factors	Always
E:	Epidemiology	Emphasising
H:	History	History-taking &
E:	Examination	Examining
P:	Pathology	Patients
I:	Investigations	In
M:	Management	Managing
C:	Complications	Clinical
P:	Prognosis	Problems

Procedures

I:	Indications
A:	Anatomy
I:	Investigations (pre-operative)
P:	Procedure
C:	Complications
P:	Prognosis

CONDITIONS

CONDITIONS

D: An abscess is a collection of pus walled off by an area of inflammation.

A: Pyogenic abscesses are caused by infection that the body's defenses have failed to completely overcome. Common bacteria include *Staphylococcus aureus*, streptococci (especially *S. pyogenes*), enteric organisms (e.g. *Escherichia coli*), other coliforms and anaerobes (e.g. *Bacteroides* spp.). TB classically causes 'cold' abscesses.

A/R: **Local:** Tissue necrosis, a closed underperfused space or foreign body that provides a focus for infection, e.g. a tooth or root fragment, splinters, mesh of hernia repairs, embedded hair, malignancy.
Systemic: Diabetes, immunosuppression (although may interfere with pus formation).

E: Common in all ages.

H: The patient may complain of local effects of pain, swelling, heat, redness and impaired function of the area where the abscess is present (*dolor, tumor, calor, rubor and functio laesa*, respectively, the Celsian features of acute inflammation) and/or systemic effects such as fever and feeling unwell

E: The above features of acute inflammation are evident at the site of the abscess. If present within an organ (e.g. liver or lung, or body cavity), localising signs may be absent, the only sign being a swinging pyrexia (caused by periodic release of microbes or inflammatory mediators into the systemic circulation), which should initiate a search for an infected collection. One old adage is that if pus is somewhere and pus is nowhere, then pus is under the diaphragm (subphrenic abscess).

P: Bacteria incite an intense acute inflammatory response with formation of pus, a collection of dead and dying neutrophils, cellular debris and bacteria, if there is resistance to phagocytosis and killing. An abscess forms as it becomes surrounded by a fibrinous exudate and granulation tissue (macrophages and fibroblasts), with subsequent collagen deposition and walling off. Cold abscesses are collections of caseating necrosis containing mycobacterium; 'cold' because there is no associated acute inflammatory response.

I: **Bloods:** FBC ($\uparrow\uparrow$ neutrophils).
Imaging: Ultrasound, CT or MRI scanning, or even ^{67}Ga white cell scanning may be used in the search for the site of a collection or abscess.
Aspiration: Pus is low in glucose and acidic. Culture of pus for organisms and sensitivity to antibiotics.

M: **Prevention:** Prophylactic antibiotics (e.g. during operations), or if given early during an infection. Often not effective once an abscess has formed.
General: Principles involved include drainage of pus, removal of necrotic and foreign material, antimicrobial cover, and correction of the predisposing cause.
Surgery: Drainage of pus is carried out by incision and drainage, with debridement of the cavity and subsequent free drainage by packing of the cavity (if superficial) or by drains (if deep).
Interventional radiology: Ultrasound or CT guidance can be used to localise and aspirate the contents of an abscess.

C: Spread may result in cellulitis (in skin) or bacteraemia with systemic sepsis. If the focus of infection is not removed, a chronic abscess or discharging sinus or fistula may form. Occasionally, antibiotics may penetrate and result in the formation of a sterile collection or antibioma. If constrained by strong facial planes, slow expansion can cause pressure necrosis of surrounding tissues.

P: Good if adequately drained and predisposing factor removed. If left untreated, abscesses tend to 'point' to the nearest epithelial surface and may spontaneously discharge their contents. Deep abscesses may become chronic, undergoing dystrophic calcification.

CONDITIONS

D: A motor disorder of the oesophagus with aperistalsis and failure of lower oesophageal sphincter relaxation while swallowing.

A: Degeneration of ganglionic cells of myenteric plexus of the oesophageal sphincter disrupts the peristaltic coordination. Cause of the degeneration is unknown. Infection with *Trypanosome cruzi* may produce a similar syndrome, but this is only common in South America.

A/R: Rare association with alacrimation and Addison's disease (Triple A syndrome).

E: Annual UK incidence is 1/100 000. All age groups but rare in childhood.

H: Intermittent dysphagia involving solids and liquids, food may be regurgitated (particularly at night), atypical/cramping retrosternal chest pain, weight loss.

E: Look for signs of complications.

P: **Micro:** Degeneration of intramural ganglionic cells of the myenteric plexus at the oesophageal sphincter. Degeneration of dorsal vagal nucleus in the brainstem medulla may also be seen.
Macro: Oesophagus can become severely dilated and elongated (see Figs 1a & 1b).

I: **CXR:** May show dilated oesophagus (double right heart border) and fluid level behind heart shadow.
Barium swallow: Dilated body of oesophagus, which smoothly tapers down to the sphincter (beak-shaped), lack of peristalsis.
Oesophagoscopy: Excludes malignancy.
Manometry: Oesophageal and sphincter pressures. Abnormal sphincter-resting pressure is > 30 mmHg.
Bloods: Exclude Chagas' disease (serology for antibodies against *Trypanosome cruzi*), blood film might detect parasites.

M: **Medical:** Nifedipine or verapamil (calcium channel antagonists) or isosorbide mononitrate as needed (for short-term relief). Endoscopic balloon dilatation of lower oesophageal sphincter (80% success rate, but small risk of perforation). Endoscopic injection of botulinum toxin may be promising.
Surgery: Heller's cardiomyotomy of lower oesophageal sphincter via an abdominal or thoracic approach to relieve obstruction. This can cause future reflux oesophagitis, so it may be combined with a fundoplication procedure.

C: If untreated, aspiration pneumonia, malnutrition and weight loss may result. 5% risk of oesophageal malignancy regardless of treatment (on average ~ 25 years after diagnosis).

P: Good if treated. If untreated, oesophageal dilation worsens, causing pressure on mediastinal structures.

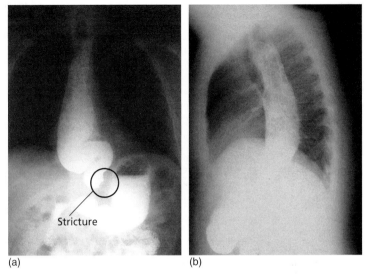

(a) (b)

Fig. 1 Achalasia: (a) AP; (b) lateral – food particles in the oesophagus.

CONDITIONS

CONDITIONS

D: Benign fibroma of the vestibulocochlear (VIII) nerve sheath. Schwannomas are often included as well.

A: The vestibulocochlear (VIII) cranial nerve sheath develops a space-occupying fibroma expanding out of the internal acoustic meatus into the cerebellopontine angle, causing compression of structures (other cranial roots and brainstem) in that region.

A/R: In type II neurofibromatosis, bilateral acoustic neuromas are associated with meningiomas, gliomas, peripheral and spinal schwannomas. There have been reports of acoustic neuroma associated with acoustic trauma, e.g. chronic exposure to loud noise.

E: Incidence is 1/100 000 per year. Occurs at all ages, more common in 40–50 years (unilateral) or 20–30 years (bilateral). Female > male. Represents 8% of all intracranial tumours in adults and 80–90% of cerebellopontine angle tumours.

H: Unilateral hearing loss, vertigo.

E: Progressive unilateral sensorineural hearing loss.
Nystagmus to the side opposite to tumour.
Larger tumours compress trigeminal (V) nerve (unilateral facial numbness), and then facial (VII) nerve (unilateral LMN facial palsy).
Look for neurofibromas at other sites.

P: Fibromas and schwannomas are the commonest growths, virtually always benign but local growth can cause serious consequences.

I: **Auditory evoked potentials:** This will show waveform delays, excluding lesions in the cochlea or the ear.
MRI: This will show the size and extent of the tumour. Gadolinium enhancement is particularly helpful to highlight the tumour clearly.

M: **Medical:** None.
Surgical: Curative treatment; however, hearing is often permanently impaired. Morbidity depends on size of tumour. Radiosurgery (stereotactic radiotherapy) may be considered for neuromas < 3 cm and in patients unfit for conventional surgery.
Advice: Patients with bilateral tumours need to learn how to lip-read and use sign language, and should start practising before curative surgery is attempted.

C: Progressive compression of brainstem, pyramidal tracts and the fourth ventricle can result from large tumours (presenting with bulbar cranial nerve palsies, reversal of the nystagmus, ipsilateral ataxia, obstruction at the level of the fourth ventricle, hydrocephalus, ↑ ICP, occipital headaches).

P: Hearing loss is often permanent. Treatment merely prevents further damage.

I: **Ischaemia, infarction or gangrene:** Acute or chronic lower limb ischaemia or caused by severe trauma or burns.

Malignancy: Certain tumours (e.g. osteosarcoma, malignant melanoma).

Severe infection: Gas gangrene (*Clostridium perfringens*) or necrotising fasciitis.

Rare: Intractable ulceration or painful paralysed limbs.

A: **Above-knee amputation (AKA):** At the level of 15 cm above the tibial plateau is optimal.

Through-knee amputation: Sometimes indicated (e.g. if there has been prior orthopaedic fixation of femur), but the disadvantage is unpredictable healing of skin flaps and a bulbous stump with difficult prosthesis fitting.

Gritti–Stokes amputation: Involves femur division at the supracondylar level, leaving a longer stump than AKA and ↑ stability for the patient while sitting.

Others (e.g. disarticulation of hip, hindquarter amputation): These are rarely performed, and mainly for severe infection or malignancy.

I: **Pre-op:** Ideally, multidisciplinary assessment including surgical, anaesthetic, prosthetic specialists. Assessment of the level of amputation given severity of disease and patient factors (e.g. rehabilitation prospects). Insulin sliding scale if diabetic, appropriate blood tests and crossmatch blood, urinary catheterisation if appropriate.

Post-op: DVT prophylaxis. Rehabilitation with early physiotherapy, early walking aids (e.g. pneumatic post-amputation mobility aid) or prosthesis fitting.

P: **Access:** Two equal fish mouth–shaped skin flaps are marked on the skin, with their upper ends at the level of femur transaction. This is 15 cm above the tibial plateau.

Muscle and vessel ligation: During skin incision, the long saphenous vein is ligated and the muscles of the anterior and posterior thigh compartments divided by diathermy. Vastus lateralis is sutured to the adductors, and quadriceps to the hamstrings. Arteries and veins are ligated and nerves divided cleanly under gentle traction.

Bone amputation: The femur is stripped of periosteum and divided, with filing of bone ends to create a smooth surface.

Closure: Once haemostasis is achieved, the two myoplastic flaps are brought together and the skin closed with interrupted sutures. A suction vacuum drain may be left in situ.

C: **Early:** Pain, DVT, flap ischaemia, stump haematoma, neuroma or infection, stump length too long or short, bony spurs, psychological problems.

Late: 'Phantom' limb pain (reduced by strong analgesia post-op), neuroma formation, erosion of bone through skin, ischaemia, osteomyelitis, ulceration. Amputations are most often carried out in those with concomitant severe atherosclerotic disease and there is a major risk of other vascular problems with survival only 30% at 5 years post-amputation.

For diagrammatic review on general amputations see Fig. 2.

PROCEDURES

Amputation, Below knee

I: **Ischaemia, infarction or gangrene:** Acute or chronic lower limb ischaemia or caused by severe trauma or burns.
Malignancy: Certain tumours (e.g. osteosarcoma, malignant melanoma).
Severe infection: Gas gangrene (*Clostridium perfringens*) or necrotising fasciitis.
Rare: Intractable ulceration or painful paralysed limbs.

A: **Below-knee:** Two techniques for transtibial amputation: Burgess long posterior flap and Robinson's skew flap techniques.
Ankle level: Seldom performed due to difficulty attaching prosthesis.
Midfoot: Lisfranc's involving disarticulation between tarsal and metatarsal bones or Chopart's disarticulation of the talonavicular and calcaneocuboid joints.
Ray: Involves excision of a toe by division through the metatarsal bone.
Toe: Division is through the proximal phalanx, as cutting through a joint exposes avascular cartilage that does not heal well.

I: **Pre-op:** Ideally, multidisciplinary assessment including surgical, anaesthetic, prosthetic specialists, physiotherapists, psychologists, etc. Assessment of the level of amputation given severity of disease and patient factors (e.g. rehabilitation prospects). Insulin sliding scale if diabetic, appropriate blood tests and crossmatch blood, urinary catheterisation if appropriate.
Post-op: DVT prophylaxis. Rehabilitation with early physiotherapy, early walking aids (e.g. pneumatic post-amputation mobility aid), prosthesis fitting.

P: **Access:** Skin flaps are marked on the skin prior to incision with a longer posterior flap (Burgess) or skew anteromedial and posterolateral flaps. The level of tibial transaction is 14 cm below knee joint or 10–12 cm below tibial tuberosity.
Ligation of muscle and vessels: During skin incision the long saphenous vein is ligated and the muscles of the anterior and peroneal compartments divided by diathermy. Arteries and veins are ligated and, following diathermy of accompanying vasa nervorum, the tibial nerve divided cleanly under gentle traction.
Bone amputation: The fibula is divided 2 cm proximally following stripping of periosteum. The tibia is also stripped and divided, with filing of bone ends to a smooth surface.
Closure: The posterior flap includes some gastrocnemius muscle to cover the cut tibia, forming a cylindrical stump. After haemostasis is achieved the skin is closed with interrupted sutures. A suction vacuum drain may be left in situ.

C: **Early:** Pain, DVT, flap ischaemia, stump haematoma, neuroma or infection, stump length too long or short, bony spurs, psychological problems.
Late: 'Phantom' limb pain (reduced by strong analgesia post-op), neuroma formation, erosion of bone through skin, ischaemia, osteomyelitis, ulceration.

P: Amputations are most often carried out in those with concomitant severe atherosclerotic disease and there is major risk of other vascular problems with survival only 30% at 5 years.
For diagrammatic review on general amputations see Fig. 2.

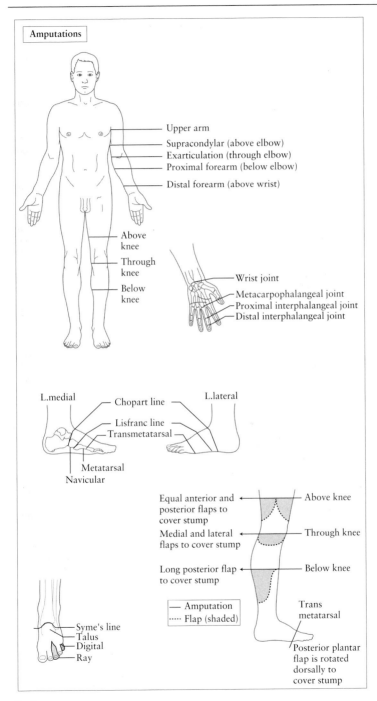

Amputations

Upper arm
Supracondylar (above elbow)
Exarticulation (through elbow)
Proximal forearm (below elbow)
Distal forearm (above wrist)

Above knee
Through knee
Below knee

Wrist joint
Metacarpophalangeal joint
Proximal interphalangeal joint
Distal interphalangeal joint

L.medial
Chopart line
L.lateral
Lisfranc line
Transmetatarsal
Metatarsal
Navicular

Equal anterior and posterior flaps to cover stump
Above knee

Medial and lateral flaps to cover stump
Through knee

Long posterior flap to cover stump
Below knee

— Amputation
···· Flap (shaded)

Trans metatarsal

Syme's line
Talus
Digital
Ray

Posterior plantar flap is rotated dorsally to cover stump

Fig. 2

Anal carcinoma

D: Malignancy arising in the anal canal

A: Linked to oncogenic types of human papilloma virus (e.g. 16, 18).

A/R: Genital warts, homosexual men and those engaging in anoreceptive intercourse may be at higher risk, HIV, chronic fistulae and previous pelvic irradiation may also ↑ risk.

E: Uncommon, 3–4% of large bowel carcinomas, females > males (but anal margin tumours more common in men), mean age 50–70 years.

H: Rectal bleeding, pruritus ani, anal discomfort, pain or discharge, tenesmus.
If there is sphincter involvement, faecal incontinence will occur.

E: An ulcer or proliferative growth may be seen on inspection of the anal margin or an area of induration or mass felt on PR examination. 15–30% will have palpable inguinal lymph nodes at presentation (but only ∼ 50% will contain tumour).

P: **Micro:** Most common type is squamous cell carcinoma (80%), remainder are adenocarcinoma or more rarely, malignant melanoma (most common site after skin and eye), and are usually unpigmented. Anal intraepithelial neoplasia describes dysplasia in the squamous epithelium with nuclear hyperchromatism, cellular and nuclear pleomorphism and abnormal mitoses and is thought to be premalignant.
Macro: Anal carcinoma is classified into two groups based on location: anal canal (tends to be poorly differentiated non-keratinising) and anal margin tumours (15–30%, tend to be well differentiated producing keratin). Tumours above the dentate line spread to pelvic lymph nodes, while those below spread to inguinal nodes.
TNM staging system: 0: carcinoma in situ; **I:** ≤ 2 cm, no sphinter involvement; **II:** ≥ 2 cm, but nodes or adjacent organs not involved; **IIIA:** spread to perirectal nodes or adjacent organs; **IIIB:** spread to iliac or inguinal nodes or adjacent organs and perirectal nodes; **IV:** spread to distant nodes/organs.

I: **Proctoscopy and biopsy:** For histology. Examination under anaesthesia may be necessary.
Bloods: FBC (for anaemia), LFT.
Imaging: Endoanal ultrasound to assess muscle invasion, MRI or CT scanning for staging. CXR to look for metastasis.

M: Combined modalities of chemotherapy and radiotherapy are used in the management of anal carcinoma, with outcomes comparable to radical surgery with preservation of the anal sphincter. Agents (e.g. 5-fluorouracil and mitomicin C or cisplatin) are used in combination with local radiotherapy to the anal area and inguinal nodes.
Surgery: Local excision of small epidermoid carcinomas of the anal margin may be curative. In the past, abdomino-perineal resection was carried out for carcinomas of the anal canal; however, with advances in chemoradiotherapy, this is now usually reserved for residual disease, recurrence post radiotherapy, those with obstructive cancers or other malignancies of the anal canal (e.g. adenocarcinoma).

C: **Local:** Pain, bleeding, incontinence, rectovaginal fistula if neglected.
From radiotherapy: Radiation-induced dermatitis, perineal irritation, proctitis and diarrhoea.

P: Important factors are histological type, site, differenciation and stage. 5 years survival for early stage squamous carcinomas treated by radical chemo/radiotherapy is 80%; if inguinal nodes are involved, this is reduced to 30%. Melanoma in this region has a poor prognosis, with only a 10% cure rate by surgery.

D: A longitudinal tear in the squamous epithelium of the distal anal canal.

A: Commonly caused by passage of a large hard stool, resulting in pain and sphincter spasm that interferes with local blood supply and hence, healing. A self-perpetuating cycle of pain, spasm and re-injury results.

A/R: Constipation.

E: Common, occurs at any age, especially 30–50 years and in children, males slightly more commonly than females.

H: Severe acute pain at the anus on defecation that may last from a few minutes to hours, often with a small amount of bleeding (seen as bright red blood streaked on the toilet paper, not mixed with stool). There is subsequent fear of defecation and constipation.

E: On inspection, the fissure is visible as a small linear cut, but is often concealed by sphincter spasm. A chronic fissure is often associated with a 'sentinel pile', which is a small skin tag present on the anal verge. Rectal examination may be aided by application of local anaesthetic but is usually not possible due to the severity of the pain.

P: The anal fissure is nearly always in the midline of the posterior anal margin extending from the anal margin to a point below the dentate line, probably because this region is a vascular watershed and susceptible to poor healing. The fissure is of variable depth with granulation tissue or fibres of the external anal sphincter visible. 10% in women and 1% in men are anterior.

I: Diagnosis is usually made on history and examination (under anaesthesia if necessary). Fissures that are not in the midline (rare) should be treated with caution and biopsied as may be due to infection (syphilitic chancre, herpes simplex, TB), IBD or malignancy.

M: **Medical:** Chemical sphincterotomy by the topical application of 0.2% glyceryl trinitrate ointment. This releases local nitric oxide that mediates smooth muscle relaxation, reducing spasm and allowing healing (major side-effect is headache). Other agents that have been shown to be effective are topical calcium channel blocker, diltiazem and injections of botulinum toxin. Pain relief is given in the form of local anaesthetic gel (1% lignocaine) applied before defecation. Laxatives may be necessary (stool softeners or bulk laxatives) to relieve straining. General advice on the avoidance of constipation should be given (e.g. a high-fibre diet, ↑ water intake and appropriate exercise).
Surgical: When there is failure of conservative treatment. Lateral submucous (internal) sphincterotomy involves division of fibres of the internal sphincter, at the 3 o'clock position, distal to the line of the anal valves. This is an effective procedure, but the patient needs to be warned about the risk of incontinence or flatus for a variable period afterwards. Anal stretches are no longer performed as it has often produced irreparable damage to the anal sphincter.

C: An abscess or a subsequent fistula may develop (see Fig. 25b). Up to 15% of those undergoing surgery will experience incontinence of flatus.

P: Generally good with glyceryl trinitrate, which is said to cure up to 60% of anal fissures, may become chronic if left untreated.

Angiodysplasia

D: Angiodysplasias are GI mucosal vascular ectasias (dilatations) that develop with ageing, most commonly occurring in the colon.

A: Exact unknown but thought to be acquired as a degenerative process, possibly resulting from chronic, low-grade obstruction of submucosal veins.

A/R: Distinction from diverticular disease can be difficult as 50% of those with bleeds secondary to angiodysplasia also have diverticular disease; has also been associated with aortic stenosis and von Willebrand's disease.

E: Present in ∼6% of those undergoing colonoscopy for variable indications and more common in elderly (∼25% in >60 years, most remaining asymptomatic).

H: Presents with bleeding PR, can be acute and rapid, characteristically intermittent with spontaneous cessation. Re-bleeding is common. The type of bleeding and volume of blood loss should be estimated.

E: Signs of shock if significant blood loss (hypotension, tachycardia).
No characteristic signs on abdominal examination.

P: **Macro:** Angiodysplasias often occur in the caecum and ascending colon, although the left colon can also be affected. On colonoscopy the lesions are visible as small, raised or flat 'cherry-red' areas. 25% of cases are multiple.
Micro: Consist of dilated tortuous thin-walled submucosal vessels that contain only small amount of muscle in their walls.

I: **Bloods:** FBC, U&Es, clotting, crossmatch (6 units if significant bleed).
Endoscopy: Proctosigmoidoscopy as part of initial assessment, upper GI endoscopy should be carried out in cases of massive haemorrhage when source unknown. Once stable and can tolerate bowel preparation, colonoscopy.
Imaging: Angiography of superior or inferior mesenteric arteries shows vascular tufts in the capillary phase and early filling of dilated veins (>1 ml/min blood loss required to visualise bleeding source). Radionucleotide scanning: ^{99m}Tc-labelled RBCs can detect bleeding of 0.5 ml/min, but lacks spatial discrimination.

M: **Emergency:** Assessment of haemodynamic status and resuscitation, O_2, IV access and fluids, blood transfusion if required. In elderly with significant bleeds, invasive monitoring may be necessary (CVP monitoring and urinary catheter).
Endoscopic: Angiodysplasias may be treated by diathermy or photocoagulation during colonoscopy.
Surgery: Need is dictated by rate and severity of blood loss. Following anterograde colon lavage by placement of a catheter in the appendix stump; on-table colonoscopy can be used to confirm the location of the bleeding and a segmental resection and primary anastomosis or a subtotal colectomy performed. If the source of bleeding is unclear, a rectal source is again excluded and on-table enteroscopy undertaken to examine for distal small bowel lesions.
Interventional radiology: Angiography and transcatheter embolisation of bleeding vessels can be used (can have serious complications, e.g. bowel ischaemia).

C: Haemorrhage, hypovolaemic shock, complications of investigations and treatment.

P: Bleeding is usually self-limiting. ∼50% of those with bleeding episodes treated conservatively with observation and transfusion will continue to have episodes during the next few years.

D: Permanent localised dilatation of the abdominal aorta greater than 3 cm.

A: 95% of AAAs are due to atherosclerosis. Other aetiologies are inflammatory (variant of atherosclerotic aneurysms), traumatic, infective (mycotic) and connective tissue diseases, Marfan's syndrome and Ehlers–Danlos type IV.

A/R: Hypertension, smoking and family history.

E: 5% of the population > 60 years and 15% > 80 years will have an AAA. Male : female is 4–6 : 1.

H: The majority are asymptomatic, may be found incidentally. Symptoms may be related to vertebral body erosion, distal embolisation, thrombosis or rupture.
Emergency presentation: May have epigastric or back pain ranging from vague discomfort to excruciating pain, or collapse associated with leakage or rupture. Rarely, present with GI bleeding due to erosion into the duodenum or high output cardiac failure due to aortocaval fistula.

E: A pulsatile mass is felt above the umbilicus. If leaking or rupture, abdominal and back tenderness with pallor, tachycardia, hypotension and hypovolaemic shock.

P: Atherosclerosis leads to thinning of the media, loss of smooth muscle cells and elastic fibres with progressive replacement by noncontractile inelastic collagen leading to generalised dilatation of the vessel. Most commonly involve the infrarenal aorta, with iliac involvement in 30% cases (see Fig. 3). Risk of rupture is related to diameter (Laplace's law: tension proportional to radius and pressure): > 5.5 cm risk 10–15% per year, if 7 cm risk is > 75%. Patients with rupture surviving until arrival in hospital usually have a leak tamponaded within the retroperitoneum.

I: **Bloods:** FBC, U&Es, clotting, crossmatch blood in acute presentation.
Imaging: CT scan or ultrasound: Confirms presence and size of the aneurysm.
Arteriography or MRA: May be necessary to measure involvement of the renal arteries prior to treatment (Figs 3a and 3b).

M: **Conservative:** Small asymptomatic aneurysms (less than 5.5 cm) are followed up with regular ultrasound and treatment for cardiovascular risk factors.
Radiological: Endovascular treatment by stent placement is increasing with trials underway to compare with standard open repairs, e.g. EVAR trials.
Surgical: AAA surgery with tube or bifurcation grafts (see Procedures).
Indications: Leaking or ruptured aneurysm – if high suspicion should be taken straight to theatre.
Asymptomatic aneurysms more than 5.5 cm in diameter.
Symptomatic aneurysms.
Expanding aneurysms (> 0.5 cm in 1 year).

C: **From disease:** Rupture (most frequent), distal embolus, sudden complete thrombosis, infection (gram-negative organisms or *staphylococci*), chronic consumptive coagulopathy, renal failure (from RAS), gut ischaemia, aortic-intestinal fistula, arteriovenous fistula from aneurysm eroding into the IVC.
From surgery: Haemorrhage, embolism, graft thrombosis, graft infection.

P: Risk of rupture related to size of aneurysm.
< 50% of patients with a ruptured AAA reach hospital alive and only about 50% of these survive (overall 80% mortality).
Elective surgery, however, have a mortality of < 5% with a 5-year survival of 72%.

CONDITIONS

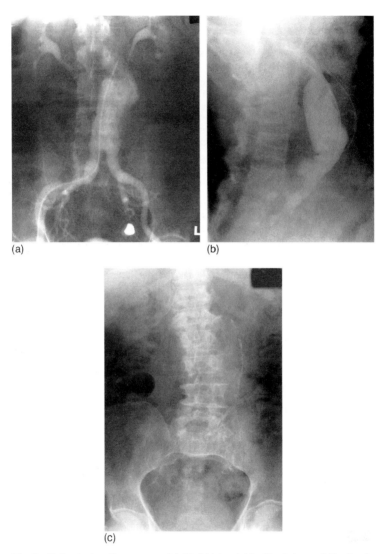

(a)

(b)

(c)

Fig. 3 Abdominal aortic aneurysm: (a) AP; (b) lateral; (c) with obvious calcification in the arterial walls.

I: **Elective:** Large asymptomatic aneurysms (> 5.5 cm in diameter). Expanding aneurysms (> 0.5 cm in 1 year). Symptomatic aneurysms.
Emergency: Leaking or ruptured aneurysms.

A: The abdominal aorta is a retroperitoneal structure entering the abdomen in front of the 12th thoracic vertebra. It descends anterior to the lumbar vertebra, dividing in front of the 4th lumbar vertebra to form the right and left common iliac arteries. The IVC, cisterna chili and the azygos vein lies on its right while the left sympathetic trunk runs close to its left margin.

I: In elective repairs, aneurysm size and anatomy is assessed by ultrasound or CT/MRA scanning.
Pre-op: FBC, clotting, U&Es, crossmatch (6–8 units of blood).
Post-op: Urinary catheter and close monitoring of fluid balance. Inspect lower limbs for emboli. DVT prophylaxis.

P: **Open AAA repair: Access:** A vertical midline laparotomy incision is made from the xiphoid to the pubis followed by abdominal exploration.
Exposure: The small bowel is displaced upwards to the right, exposing the retroperitoneum over the aorta, which is incised slightly to the right to prevent damage to the left sympathetic chain. Dissection is carried out to expose the aorta from the infrarenal aorta to the bifurcation, with care taken to avoid injury to the left renal vein, which crosses in front of the aorta. The inferior mesenteric artery is identified, ligated and transected. Systemic heparin is administered and clamps are placed at the proximal and distal ends of the aneurysm.
Opening the aneurysm: The aneurysm is opened longitudinally, exposing the contents. Thrombus within the aneurysm is removed, and any bleeding from lumbar arteries in the back wall controlled with sutures.
Insertion of graft: The walls of the distal aorta and bifurcation are inspected. In an aneurysm confined to the aorta, a tube graft is used. If the distal aorta or proximal iliacs are diseased, an aorto-iliac or more rarely, aorto-bifemoral trouser graft is used. The grafts are sutured in place with Prolene sutures and flushed to remove air or debris.
Assessment of graft: The aortic clamp is gradually released ensuring haemostasis, followed by gradual opening of the distal end with close monitoring due to the risk of hypotension and arrythmias. The aneurysm sac is then closed around the graft and sutured to prevent adhesions with the anastomosis suture line.
Closure: 3-layer closure with one continuous suture for all deep layers, one continuous suture for subcuticular fat, and staples, subcuticular or interrupted sutures for the skin.
Post-op care is usually within an ITU or HDU setting with close monitoring. In emergency setting of aneurysm rupture, the patient is rushed to theatre, maintaining systolic BP of ~80–100 mmHg. Following 'crash' induction of anaesthesia, the patient is rapidly draped, prepared with aim for rapid clamping and control of the bleeding vessel.

C: Haemorrhage, myocardial ischaemia, MI or arrhythmias, CVA, respiratory complications (atelectasis, infection, ARDS), colonic ischaemia, spinal ischaemia, atheromatous embolisation, renal failure, graft thrombosis, endoleak. Late: graft infection, aorto-enteric fistula, false aneurysm at anastomosis.

P: Elective operative mortality is now < 5% in most units. Emergency repair of a leaking or ruptured aortic aneurysm has a very high mortality.

Aortic dissection

D: Aortic dissection occurs when a tear in the artery intima allows blood to enter the media, separating the inner and outer layers producing a false channel.
Stanford classification**:** Type A involving the ascending ($+/-$descending) aorta; type B involving only the descending aorta.
De Bakey classification**:** Type I: proximal tear, with dissection involving ascending and descending aorta; type II: ascending aorta only; type III: descending aorta only.

A: Caused by a defect in the artery intima and weakness of the media in association with risk factors mentioned below.

A/R: Hypertension, atherosclerosis, Marfan's syndrome, tertiary syphillis, rarely iatrogenic injury during arteriography.

E: Uncommon, but often lethal. Male > female, peak incidence in 50–70 years.

H: Sudden, very severe chest pain ('tearing' in quality) that radiates through to the back, no prodromal symptoms.

E: Hypertension (but if rupture occurs, shock develops); heart murmur (early diastolic) may be present due to the acute aortic regurgitation.
In some patients there are unequal limb pulses (measure BP in both arms) or signs of an acute CVA due to occlusion of the main vessels off the aortic arch.

P: $\frac{2}{3}$ occur in the anterior wall above the aortic valve and $\frac{1}{3}$ on the posterior wall of the proximal descending aorta (sites of maximal stress). Occasionally, the tract can re-enter the main lumen, creating a 'double-barrelled' aorta. In some cases there is cystic medial necrosis, a form of mucoid degeneration of the media with elastic fibre fragmentation; an exaggerated form of this is present in Marfan's disease.

I: **CXR:** Widened mediastinum (but normal in up to 50%), occasionally a left pleural effusion occurs with a contained rupture.
CT scan: Can be used for rapid diagnosis.
MRA, echocardiography (transoesophageal): Can give information about valve competence.
ECG: As 10% will develop an MI due to retrograde dissection of the ascending aorta, resulting in occlusion of the right coronary artery.

M: **Medical:** Suitable for uncomplicated distal or stable arch dissection. Aggressive control of BP (e.g. with sodium nitroprusside or β-blockers) to prevent extension of the dissection. Close monitoring of vital signs.
Surgical: Treatment of choice for proximal dissection and distal dissection with organ compromise, rupture or impending rupture. Involves resection of the ascending aorta and replacement with a synthetic graft. If the aortic root is involved, the aortic valve is replaced with reimplantation of the coronary ostia (Bentall procedure).

C: Acute aortic regurgitation, MI, cardiac tamponade, stroke, renal failure, spinal cord or bowel ischaemia. Initial diagnostic error, delay in referral for surgery or tear perpetuation by administration of thrombolytics for misdiagnosis of AMI is not uncommon.

P: **Type A:** >80% mortality without surgery, falling to 20% with surgery.
Type B: Mortality is lower, but up to 20% of survivors will develop an AAA and imaging surveillance is recommended.

I: Acute appendicitis.

A: The appendix, a vestigial organ, arises at the convergence of the taeniae coli on the posteromedial side of the caecum, 2.5 cm below the junction with the terminal ileum. The length varies from 1.2–22.0 cm and the appendix can lie in variable positions, retrocaecal (∼70%), pelvic (20%), subcaecal (2%) and pre- or post-ileal (5%). It has a mesentery, the mesoappendix, in which runs the appendicular artery, a branch of the ileocolic artery. Lymphatics from the appendix traverse the mesoappendix to drain into ileocaecal nodes.

I: **Pre-op:** FBC, U&Es, LFT, amylase, CRP, urinalysis. In females of childbearing age, a pregnancy test should be performed. Antibiotic prophylaxis is given.
Post-op: Antibiotics may be continued if the appendix is inflamed.

P: **Access:** Lanz (transverse skin crease) incision is made 2 cm below the umbilicus, centred on the midclavicular–midinguinal line, the SC fat divided and external oblique aponeurosis exposed. A small slit is made in the direction of the fibres of the external oblique, then extended with scissors. Internal oblique muscle is split along the direction of its fibres by blunt dissection, as is transversus and the opening gently enlarged using retractors. Once the peritoneum is exposed, it is gently picked up with a clip. A second clip is then placed and the first clip repositioned. The length between the clips is palpated (for any bowel caught up between the clips) before a small cut is made, and then extended.
Identification: The caecum is identified and the taeniae followed to find the base of the appendix, freeing it from inflammatory adhesions by gentle blunt dissection. Babcock's forceps is used to pick up the appendix. If the appendix is found to be normal ('lily-white'), it should still be removed; however, the small bowel should be systematically inspected for terminal ileitis, a Meckel's diverticulum or mesenteric adenitis. In females, the right ovary and tube should be inspected.
Resection: The mesoappendix is clipped and divided after tying off, ensuring haemostasis. A crushing clamp is used to crush the base of the appendix and a tie placed around the base before removal. The appendix is sent for histological analysis. Usually the appendix stump is buried using a purse string suture. The cavity should be washed if there has been inflammatory fluid or pus.
Closure: The incision is then closed in layers. A continuous suture of the peritoneum, interrupted sutures to the muscle layers and then continuous sutures to the external oblique (the latter is very important in preventing subsequent hernias) are performed. A subcuticular absorbable suture is usually used for the skin. Local anaesthetic infiltration reduces post-op pain.
Laparoscopic appendicectomy: An alternative technique, which is very useful in women where the diagnosis may be equivocal as it can be both diagnostic and therapeutic.

C: Relatively uncommon, but presence reflects the degree of inflammation or peritonitis (e.g. ileus, haemorrhage, wound infection, more rarely, local abscess or a pelvic abscess).

P: Usually good with mortality < 1% but this can be higher in elderly or if perforation occurs.

Appendicitis

D: Acute inflammation and infection of the appendix.

A: Thought to be initiated by luminal obstruction by a faecolith (inspissated faeces), lymphoid hyperplasia or oedema.

A/R: May be associated with low dietary fibre intake.

E: Any age, but most common in < 40 years. Appendicectomy is one of the most common emergency surgical operation, with about 1/6 lifetime risk.

H: **Classic presentation** (< 50% of cases): Abdominal pain (usually < 72 h), initially diffuse, periumbilical and colicky (visceral pain lasting a few hours). The pain becomes sharp and localised to the RIF (somatic pain as parietal peritoneum involved). Anorexia (the most constant symptom) and nausea are common. Vomiting may develop hours after onset of pain.
Alternative presentations: Pain in the right flank (retrocaecal appendix), the right upper quadrant (long appendix) or lower abdomen (pelvic appendix). May be associated urinary frequency or loose stools due to bladder or bowel irritation by the inflamed appendix.

E: Mild pyrexia, facial flush, tachycardia.
Abdominal pain often maximal at McBurney's point (2/3 along a line from the umbilicus to the anterior superior iliac spine) with rebound tenderness (demonstrable on percussion) and guarding.
Signs of peritoneal inflammation: pain on coughing or while sucking in or blowing out the abdominal wall.
Rovsing's sign is pain in the RIF elicited by pressure over the LIF, but is unreliable.

P: Luminal obstruction results in proliferation of bowel flora and inflammation that extends transmurally. Swelling results in obstruction and thrombosis of end arteries and the appendix becomes gangrenous and necrotic. The inflammation may become localised by omentum or bowel loops to form an appendix mass or abscess, or perforation and spreading peritonitis may occur if not treated.

I: Appendicitis is a clinical diagnosis; there is no definitive test to confirm or exclude it.
Bloods: ↑ WCC and CRP (especially in later stages), amylase (to exclude pancreatitis), U&Es.
Urine: For microscopy, culture and sensitivity (to exclude infection), pregnancy test in women of childbearing age.
Imaging: AXR or ultrasound (not usually diagnostic).

M: **General:** Rehydration with IV fluids, broad-spectrum antibiotics are given pre- and peri-op (e.g. cefuroxime and metronidazole). If symptoms or signs are equivocal, observation with frequent re-examination.
Surgery: Appendicectomy (see Procedures). In young women, diagnostic laparoscopy may be necessary if diagnosis is not certain.
Post-op, antibiotics may be given for up to 48 h in early cases but for 7–10 days in cases of gangrenous or perforated appendix. If an **appendix abscess** is present, drainage must be performed, either percutaneously with ultrasound control or intra-operatively (with appendicectomy if safe). Management of an **appendiceal mass** may be non-operative with antibiotics, parenteral fluids and frequent reassessment, with operation if clinical deterioration occurs. Interval appendicectomy performed 6–8 weeks later (Ochsner–Sherren approach). If this is not performed in adults, imaging such as barium enema or colonocopy should be done to exclude a local perforation, e.g. of carcinoma of the right colon.

C: Formation of an inflammatory mass, appendix abscess, perforation and peritonitis, rarely portal pyemia.

Post-op: Wound infection, wound abscess, abdominal abscess, adynamic ileus, rarely a faecal fistula from the appendix stump.

P: Appendicectomy is curative. If untreated, it can be life-threatening. Diagnosis is difficult in the very young, elderly and in pregnancy; morbidity and mortality in those groups are higher.

CONDITIONS

Arteriovenous fistulae and malformations

D: An arteriovenous fistula or malformation is an abnormal communication between an artery and vein that bypasses the capillary bed.

A: **Congenital:** Fistulae can be divided into *haemangiomas*, e.g strawberry naevi, and *malformations* (AVMs). The latter is divided into *low flow* or *high flow* (e.g. hepatic or pulmonary AVM).
Acquired: Trauma, tumours (e.g. glomus tumour, hepatoma, hypernephroma and sarcomas), infection, inflammation (e.g. aortocaval fistula) or iatrogenic (e.g. Brescia–Cimino fistula for haemodialysis or portocaval shunt in portal hypertension).

A/R: AVMs are associated with many different syndromes, e.g. Klippel–Trénaunay, Kasabach–Merritt, Sturge–Weber, von-Hippel–Lindau and Rendu–Osler–Weber syndrome (the latter is caused by a defect in the protein, endoglin, which carries a 30% risk of developing a pulmonary AVM).

E: AVMs such as cutaneous haemangiomas are common, the others less so.

H: Presentation is variable, depending on the site and size of the AVM and symptoms may be due to local, peripheral or systemic effects (see below). Congenital AVMs involving the skin are often visible from birth (haemangiomas appear $\sim$4 weeks after birth). Malformations usually grow with age, often during puberty or pregnancy in women, and those within internal organs may only be detected once complications develop; e.g. brain AVMs may cause haemorrhage, epilepsy or a neurological deficit. Other presentations include varicose veins, limb swelling or pain.

E: Cutaneous haemangiomas are usually scarlet in colour, firm and cannot be emptied of blood on compression. Internal AVMs may be revealed by an overlying bruit, possibly with reduced distal pulses and an ↑ pulse pressure. There may be signs of cardiac failure in large AVMs. There may be focal neurological signs in cerebral AVMs, especially after a complication such as haemorrhage.

P: Congenital AVMs are thought to arise due to anomalous embryonic vascular development and can involve arteries, veins, capillaries or lymphatics. Haemangiomas result from endothelial hyperplasia and contain abundant mast cells, whereas endothelial cells in malformations demonstrate normal turnover.

I: **Imaging** of the AVM can be carried out by Duplex scanning, CT or MRI scanning or invasively, by angiography.
Other: Quantification of AV shunting can be carried out using ^{99m}Tc-human albumin microspheres. These are introduced into an artery and are too large to pass through capillaries. Those passing through AVMs are trapped in the lungs and quantified using gamma camera.

M: **Conservative:** Cutaneous haemangiomas usually undergo spontaneous regression at the end of the first year of life.
Interventional radiology: In the case of internal AVMs, using metal coils or tissue adhesive or particles to embolise the AVM.
Surgery: Often difficult, but excision (after pre-op embolisation) may be possible in the case of small and accessible AVMs. Stereotactic radiosurgery using a gamma knife has been used on small brain AVMs, but takes 2 years for full effect.

C: Depends on size and location.
Local: Cosmetic disfigurement, ulceration, bleeding, local pressure, hydrocephalus.
Distal: Ischaemia of peripheral tissues,
Systemic: High-ouput cardiac failure in the case of large AVMs.

P: Depends on site and aetiology. 90% of haemangiomas regress by 5–10 years. 1–4% annual risk of haemorrhage in cerebral AVMs.

D: Commonest form of skin malignancy; also known as a 'rodent ulcer'.

A: Prolonged sun exposure or UV radiation.

A/R: Multiple basal cell carcinomas are associated with Gorlin's syndrome (naevoid basal cell carcinoma syndrome). Risk factors include photosensitising pitch, tar and oils that act as co-carcinogens to UV radiation; previous treatment with arsenic (once present in many tonics) predisposes to multiple basal cell carcinomas developing even after a lag of many years.

E: Common in geographic areas with high sunlight exposure, especially in those with fair skin, common in the elderly, rare before the age of 40 years.

H: A chronic slowly progressive skin lesion usually on the face but also on the scalp, ears or trunk.

E: **Nodulo-ulcerative** (most common): Small glistening translucent skin over a coloured papule that slowly enlarges (early) or a central ulcer ('rodent ulcer') with raised pearly edges (late). Fine telangiectatic vessels often run over the tumour surface. Cystic change may be seen in larger more protuberant lesions.
Morphoeic: Slowly expanding, yellow/white waxy plaque with an ill-defined edge.
Superficial: Most often on trunk, multiple pink/brown scaly plaques with a fine 'whipcord' edge expanding slowly; can grow to more than 10 cm in diameter.
Pigmented: Specks of brown or black pigment may be present in any type of basal cell carcinoma in all or part of the tumour.

P: Small dark blue staining basal cells growing in well-defined aggregates invading the dermis with the outer layer of cells arranged in palisades. Numerous mitotic and apoptotic bodies are seen. Growth rate is usually slow but steady and insidious. It does not metastasise, but has the potential to invade and destroy local tissues.

I: Biopsy (diagnosis is based mainly on clinical suspicion).

M: **Cryotherapy, curettage, cauterisation and photodynamic therapy** are used for small superficial lesions.
Surgical: Excision with a 0.5 cm margin of surrounding normal skin for discrete nodular or cystic nodules in patients under 60 years; Mohs' micrographic surgery, which includes careful review of tissue excised under frozen section, is the treatment of choice for large tumours (1 cm diameter) and lesions near the eyes, nose and ears. Excision and skin flap coverage may be necessary.
Radiotherapy: Useful in basal cell carcinomas involving structures that are difficult to surgically reconstruct (e.g. eyelids, tearducts). Repeated treatments may be necessary as there is risk of side-effects such as radiation dermatitis, ulceration, depilation.

C: The tumour has a slow but relentless course. Can become disfiguring on the face. Has the potential to invade into underlying cartilage and facial or skull bones and damaging important surrounding structures or eroding into blood vessels.

P: Good with appropriate treatment. If left may continue to grow, invade and ulcerate. Regular follow-up is necessary to detect local recurrence or other lesions.

CONDITIONS

Benign breast disease

D: Breast tissue changes ranging from normal to abnormal, either in development, cyclical change or involution phases. Includes fibrocystic change, breast cysts, fibroadenomas, sclerosing adenosis, intraductal papillomas, duct ectasia, periductal mastitis and fat necrosis.

A: Related to changes in response to hormones or unknown factors.
Fat necrosis occurs secondary to trauma, which causes rupture of fat cells.

A/R: May be less common in those on OCP. Smoking is a risk factor for periductal mastitis.

E: Very common. Diffuse fibrocystic changes are very common, being seen in as many as 60% of women, and 70% experience mastalgia. Fibroadenomas are more common in 15–35 years.

H: History of breast discomfort or pain (cyclical or noncyclical mastalgia), swelling or lump. Nipple discharge (if bloodstained, malignancy should be suspected). Risk factors for breast cancer should be ascertained including family history, menstrual history, pregnancies, use of OCP or hormone replacement therapy.

E: Focal or diffuse nodularity of breasts.
Fibroadenomas are usually smooth, well circumscribed and mobile lumps ('breast mouse'). Yellow/green nipple discharge (duct ectasia).
Features of malignancy are absent, e.g. dimpling, peau d'orange skin changes, enlarged axillary lymph nodes.

P: ANDI classification maps benign conditions between normality, through benign disorders to benign breast disease.
Fibroadenoma: Result from hypertrophy of a breast lobule, contains both epithelial and connective tissue elements. There may also be apocrine hyperplasia.
Fat necrosis: Irregular adipocytes with intervening pink amorphous material and inflammatory cells, including foreign body giant cells responding to the necrotic fat cells, often mimics malignancy. Sclerosing adenosis is an aberration of normal involution. Duct ectasia is when central ducts become dilated with ductal secretion; this may leak into periductal tissues and cause an inflammatory reaction (periductal mastitis).

I: Usually performed in the context of triple assessment:
1. **Clinical examination.**
2. **Imaging:** Mammography (craniocaudal and oblique mediolateral views) or USG in younger patients (< 35 years). Benign masses are less likely to be calcified (microcalcifications are highly suggestive of malignancy).
3. **Cytology/histology:** By FNA cytology or trucut or excision biopsy.

M: **Conservative:** Symptomatic treatment, e.g. analgesia, evening primrose oil (a rich source of gammalinoleic acid) for mastalgia. Advice on wearing supportive bra and diet (that is rich in PUFA are thought to suppress hormone interaction with breast tissue). Danazol is used as second-line treatment. Fibroadenomas may be treated conservatively or removed if large or on request.
Surgery: Includes removal or excision biopsy of breast lump; a wide local excision shoud be performed if there is any suspicion that it is not benign. Microdochectomy is performed for intraductal papillomas. Hadfield's (or Adair's) operation excises central ducts in duct ectasia.

C: Pain, recurrence.

P: Good, although recurrence is common.

D: Slowly progressive nodular hyperplasia of the periurethral (transitional) zone of the prostate gland, the most frequent cause of LUTS in adult males.

A: Precise unknown but thought to be related to hormonal changes, in particular fluctuating levels of androgens and oestrogens.

A/R: A diet rich in soya and vegetables may reduce the risk and there is a negative association with cirrhosis.

E: Common, 70% of men aged 70 years have histological BPH, with 50% of these experiencing significant symptoms, West > Far East, Afrocarribean > Caucasian.

H: **Obstructive symptoms:** Hesitancy, poor or intermittent stream, terminal dribbling and incomplete emptying.
Irritative/storage symptoms: Frequency, urgency, urge incontinence and nocturia.
Acute retention: Sudden inability to pass urine, associated with severe pain.
Chronic retention: Painless, there is often frequency with passage of small volumes of urine, especially at night.

E: On digital rectal examination, the prostate is often enlarged; however, there is poor correlation between the size and symptoms and if nodular, prostate carcinoma should be suspected.
Acute retention: Suprapubic pain and a distented palpable bladder.
Chronic retention: A large distended painless bladder (residual volumes > 1 L) and there may be signs of renal failure.

P: **Micro:** From middle age, hyperplasia of the para-urethral glands with associated smooth muscle and fibrous tissue growth occurs, surrounded by a false capsule of compressed peripheral zone glandular tissue.

I: **Bloods:** U&Es for impaired renal function, PSA.
Midstream urine: For microscopy, culture and sensitivity.
Imaging: Ultrasound imaging of the renal tract to check for dilatation of the upper urinary tract. Bladder scanning to measure pre- and postvoiding volumes. TRUS to measure prostate size and guide biopsies. Flexible cystoscopy to visualise the bladder outlet and bladder changes (e.g. trabeculation).
Other: Urinary flow studies (flowmetry).

M: Depends on the severity of symptoms and the presence of complications.
Emergency: In acute retention, urinary catheterisation.
Conservative: If mild, 'watchful waiting' may be appropriate with symptom monitoring using the IPSS questionnaire.
Medical: Selective α-blockers relax smooth muscle of the internal (bladder neck) sphincter and the prostate capsule (e.g. alfuzosin, tamsulosin). 5α-reductase inhibitors act by inhibiting conversion of testosterone to dihydrotestosterone (e.g. finasteride), reduce prostate size by ~ 20%, but may take time to show improvement.
Surgery: TURP involves electrocautery-mediated resection from within the prostatic urethra. Open prostatectomy (retropubic or suprapubic approaches) is usually reserved for very large glands (> 60 g).

C: Recurrent urinary infections, acute or chronic urinary retention, urinary stasis and bladder diverticulae or stone development, obstructive renal failure, post-obstructive diuresis.
From TURP: Retrograde ejaculation (common), haemorrhage (primary, reactionary or secondary 2–10%), clot retention, more rarely incontinence, TUR syndrome (seizures or cardiovascular collapse caused by hypervolaemia and hyponatraemia due to absorption of glycine irrigation fluid), urinary infection, erectile dysfunction; late: urethral stricture.

P: Mild symptoms may be improved by medical therapies but those with marked symptoms usually obtain significant relief from surgical intervention.

CONDITIONS

D: Malignancy of bladder cells.

A: Unknown, common genetic abnormalities are chromosome 9 deletions in superficial tumours and p53 mutations and 14q or 17q deletions in more invasive tumours.

A/R: Strong association with smoking, also exposure to carcinogens such as naphthylamines and benzidine in dye, rubber and leather industries, cyclophosphamide treatment (10% risk after 12 years of exposure), pelvic irradiation (e.g. for cervical carcinoma), chronic UTIs, schistosomiasis.

E: ~ 2% of cancers, 2nd most common cancer of the genitourinary system, males 2–3× as commonly affected as women, peak incidence in 50–70 years.

H: Most commonly, painless macroscopic haematuria. Other symptoms may include urinary frequency, urgency or nocturia (irritative), recurrent UTIs. Rarely, pain due to clot retention, ureteral obstruction or extention to pelvis.

E: Often no signs. Under anaesthetic, bimanual examination is a part of disease staging.

P: **Micro:** Majority are transitional cell carcinoma, rarely squamous cell associated with chronic inflammation (e.g. in schistosomiasis), or adenocarcinomas can arise in the urachal remnant, mesenchymal tumours (e.g. leiomyosarcomas) are very rare.
Macro: Visible on cystoscopy: carcinoma in situ as an erythematous area, tumours as exophytic papillary fronds. Tends to be multifocal.
TNM staging: Tis flat carcinoma in situ, Ta papillary tumour above the lamina propria, T1 submucosal invasion of lamina propria, T2 invasion of muscle, T3 invasion of perivesical tissue, T4 invasion of adjacent organs or pelvic wall, N: nodal involvement, M: metastases.
Grading: G1 well, G2 moderately and G3 poorly differentiated.

I: **Cystoscopy:** Allows visualisation of the tumour, biopsy or removal.
USS, IVU: To assess upper and lower urinary tract, as tumours can be multifocal (see Fig. 4).
CT or MRI scan: For staging.
Other: Urine cytology, there are no consistent tumour markers associated.

M: Depends on stage and grade of tumour:
Superficial tumours (Tis, T1): TURBT. Intravesical chemotherapy with mitomycin C or intravesical immunotherapy with BCG instillation to reduce recurrence rates. Close follow-up with repeat cystoscopy and bladder cytology every 3 months for 2 years, then every 6 months for 2 years, then yearly. High-grade T1 tumours may be best treated by cystectomy.
Invasive tumours (T2 and above): Radical cystectomy if localised (includes hysterectomy and bilateral salpingo-oopherectomy in women, cystoprostatectomy in men with urinary diversion by an ileal conduit or orthoptic reconstruction. Radical radiotherapy is an alternative if unfit for surgery, with salvage cystectomy for relapse post radiotherapy. Palliative radiotherapy +/− chemotherapy is used in metastatic disease, e.g. M-VAC. (methotrexate, vinblastine, doxorubicin and cisplatin).

C: Haematuria and clot retention, hydronephrosis due to ureteric orifice obstruction.
From treatment: Postradiotherapy cystitis, haemorrhage, bladder contraction, with urinary diversion: nephrolithiasis.

P: Following TURBT, 75% will develop other tumours, only 10% progress to invasive disease. 5-year survival for T1 90–100%, T2 55%, T3 35%, T4 10–20%. Presence of nodes 6% or metastases 0%.

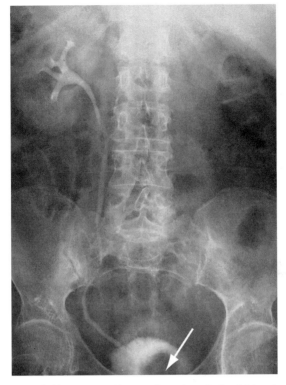

Fig. 4 Bladder tumour with a standing column in the right ureter.

Branchial cyst, sinus and fistula

D: Neck swelling or discharge that arises at the site of an embryonic pharyngeal pouch.

A: Probably arise from congenital remnants of the 2nd pharyngeal pouch or branchial cleft, although the precise embryological origin is disputed.

A/R: Occasionally associated with 1st or more rarely 3rd/4th cleft cysts.

E: Branchial cysts are the most common, presenting most often in the third decade, with considerable variation, and in men slightly more often than women.

H: Patient complains of a lateral neck swelling ($\frac{2}{3}$ left-sided) that may vary in size over time, it is usually painless unless inflammation and infection develop, then becomes painful and red. A sinus or fistula presents with a neck dimple that discharges mucus or mucopurulent fluid.

E: If this is a cyst, a lump is present just deep to sternocleidomastoid at the junction of its upper and lower $\frac{2}{3}$.
On palpation the swelling is usually ovoid, smooth and firm or may be relatively soft in early stages, fluctuant and may transilluminate. 2% are bilateral.
The external opening of a branchial sinus or fistula is at the junction of the middle and lower $\frac{1}{3}$ of the anterior edge of sternocleidomastoid.

P: Grooves in the neck, known as branchial clefts, with the intervening branchial arches appear in the 5th week of foetal development. The 1st cleft persists as the external auditory meatus, but the remainder normally disappear. If remnants of the 2nd cleft remain, a cyst, sinus or fistula may develop slowly over years. The cysts are lined by squamous epithelium and contain collections of turbid fluid consisting of epithelial debris and cholesterol crystals, and some contain lymphoid tissue.
A fistula passes between the internal and external carotid arteries, superior to the hypoglossal nerve and inferior to the glossopharyngeal nerve terminating in the posterior part of the tonsillar fossa in the oropharynx.

I: **Imaging:** Ultrasound or CT scanning can be used to visualise the cyst.
FNA is used to distinguish a branchial cyst from cervical lymph node metastases in older individuals (e.g. thyroid cancer and mucoepidermoid carcinomas of salivary glands that may have a significant cystic component).

M: **Surgery:** Treatment is surgical excision of the cyst and any associated sinus or tract. This is usually performed via a transverse neck incision. Platysma is divided and sternomastoid is retracted posteriorly to obtain access to the cyst. It is then removed by careful blunt dissection with identification and avoiding nerve damage (especially the hypoglossal and spinal accessory nerve). A branchial cyst abscess should first be drained and antibiotics given to eliminate infection before the cyst is excised.

C: Infection, branchial cyst abscess, nerve damage during surgery, incomplete excision of a sinus or fistula tract.

P: Good, with cure following complete excision.

D: Abscess formation in breast tissues.
Two main forms are recognised: puerperal (lactational) and nonpuerperal.

A: Infection. Lactational: most commonly with *Staphylococcus aureus,* nonpuerperal: *S. aureus* and anaerobes, often enterococci or bacteroides spp. (TB and actinomycosis are extremely rare causes).

A/R: Main risk factor: lactation, with bacteria gaining access through cracked nipples. Nonpuerperal: smoking, mammary duct ectasia/periductal mastitis, an associated inflammatory breast cancer should be excluded. Also associated with wound infections after breast surgery, diabetes and steroid therapy.

E: Lactational breast abscesses are common and tend to occur soon after starting breastfeeding and on weaning, when incomplete emptying of the breast results in stasis and engorgement. Nonlactational abscesses are more common in those aged 30–60 years and smokers.

H: The patient complains of breast discomfort and the development of painful swelling in an area of the breast. She may complain of feeling unwell and feverish.
Women with a nonpuerperal abscess often have a history of previous infections and systemic upset is less pronounced.

E: **Local:** Area of breast is swollen, warm, tender and the overlying skin may be inflamed; examination of the nipple may reveal cracks or fissures. In non-puerperal cases there may be evidence of scars or tissue distortion from previous episodes, or signs of duct ectasia, e.g. nipple retraction.
Systemic: Pyrexia, tachycardia.

P: **Micro:** See Abscesses.
Macro: Breast abscesses are frequently loculated. Nonpuerperal tend to arise in periareolar tissues and are often a manifestation of duct ectasia/periductal mastitis.

I: **Imaging:** Ultrasound.
Microbiology: Microscopy, culture and sensitivity of pus samples.

M: **Medical:** Early, cellulitic phase may be treated with antibiotics (flucloxacillin in the case of lactational, with the addition of metronidazole in nonpuerperal abscesses).
Surgical: *Lactational*: Daily needle aspiration with antibiotic cover may be successful, but in most cases, formal incision and drainage is carried out. Incision should allow full drainage and be cosmetically acceptable; loculi are explored and broken down with a finger. The wound may be packed lightly with anti-septic soaked kaltostat and left open, with daily packing, or primary closure performed with antibiotic cover. Breastfeeding should continue from the non-affected breast and the affected side emptied either manually or with a breast pump. Advice on avoiding cracked nipples.
Non-puerperal: Open drainage should be avoided, or carried out through a small incision. Definitive treatment should be carried out once the infection has settled by the excision of the involved duct system.

C: Mammary fistula formation, rarely overlying skin undergoes necrosis.

P: If untreated, a breast abscess will eventually point and spontaneously discharge onto the skin surface. Nonpuerperal abscesses tend to recur.

CONDITIONS

Breast carcinoma

D: Malignancy of breast tissue.

A: Combination of genetic and environmental factors. BRCA-1 (17q) and BRCA-2 (13q) gene mutations are implicated in 2% of cases.

A/R: Age, prolonged exposure to female sex hormones (particularly oestrogen), nulliparity, early menarche, late menopause and obesity. Family history is an important risk factor (5–10% cases).

E: Vying for the commonest cancer in women with lifetime risk of 1 : 9 in the UK. Peak incidence in 40–70-year-olds. Rare in men (< 1% of all breast cancers).

H: Breast lump (usually painless) or changes in breast shape.
Nipple discharge or axillary lump.
Symptoms of malignancy: Weight loss, bone pain, paraneoplastic syndromes.

E: Breast lump (usually hard, irregular, may be fixed).
Peau d'orange appearance of skin, skin tethering, fixed to chest wall.
Skin ulceration, nipple inversion.
Examine axillary nodes for lymphatic spread.
Paget's disease of the nipple: Eczematous, ulcerated, discharging nipple. This is ductal carcinoma in situ infiltrating the nipple.

P: **Histology:** *In situ carcinoma*: Ductal or lobular carcinoma in situ.
Invasive: Most common is ductal carcinoma or no special type.
Others: Lobular (10–15%), mucinous, medullary papillary, adenoid cystic, tubular and Paget's disease of the nipple.
Grading: The Nottingham modification of Bloom and Richardson grading system is a prognostic indicator. Three features assessed are tubule formation, nuclear size/pleomorphism and number of mitoses. Scores are used to generate Grade 1 (well-differentiated) to 3 (poorly differentiated).
Staging: Include Manchester staging and UICC TNM staging system:
Tumour Size (T): T1: < 2 cm T3: > 5 cm
T2: 2–5 cm T4: Any size with chest wall or skin extension
Nodes (N): N1: Mobile ipsilateral axillary
N2: Fixed ipsilateral axillary
N3: Ipsilateral internal mammary nodes
Metastases (M): M0: No distant metastases
M1: Distant metastases

I: **Triple assessment:** Standardised approach to investigating a breast lump, consisting of clinical examination, imaging (mammography or ultrasound) and tissue diagnosis (cytology or biopsy).
Mammogram: See Fig. 5. Useful screening investigation of women > 35 years. In the UK, screening begins after the age of 50 in women. Features of malignancy include branching or linear microcalcifications.
Ultrasound: To identify benign cystic lesions from sinister solid lesions. More useful in women < 35 years.
Fine-needle aspiration: Minimally invasive. This allows cytology of discrete breast lumps, and drainage of cysts.
Trucut needle biopsy: Core biopsy with a spring-loaded firing device with a wide-bore needle. This allows for a histological diagnosis.
Sentinel lymph node biopsy: Radioactive tracer is injected into the tumour and a nuclear scan identifies the sentinel node and the node is biopsied to detect spread.
Staging: CXR, liver ultrasound. Consider isotope bone scan, CT (brain or thorax).
Bloods: FBC, U&Es, Ca^{2+}, bone profile, LFT, ESR.

M: **Multidisciplinary management:** With input of breast surgeon, radiologist, oncologist, breast care nurses and consideration of individual patient's wishes.

CONDITIONS

Surgical (see Procedures):

Wide local excision/segmental mastectomy: Evidence suggests that long-term survival is similar after either mastectomy or wide local excision and radiotherapy. Smaller tumours may need radiological wire localisation pre-op. Surgery to the axilla is necessary for node staging and ranges from node sampling, e.g. sentinel node biopsy, to level III clearance (lymph nodes up past pectoralis minor to subclavius).

Modified radical mastectomy (Patey mastectomy) or segmental mastectomy: Removal of breast, surrounding fascia and axillary node clearance, but pectoralis major and pectoralis minor are preserved.

Radical mastectomy (Halstead): Very rarely performed now. Removal of breast, pectoralis major and minor and axillary node clearance.

Reconstruction: May be performed concurrently with surgical excision. Latissimus dorsi or transverse rectus abdominis myocutaneous flap are used.

Systemic therapy:

Chemotherapy: Used in premenopausal women, rapidly progressive disease, visceral involvement, oestrogen receptor negative tumours and where hormonal treatment has failed. Many regimen options (e.g. 5-fluorouracil, cyclophosphamide, methotrexate, adriamycin) with response rates in ~50% using a combination of drugs. A promising new agent is herceptin, a monoclonal antibody against HER-2 protein (tumour cell growth promoter).

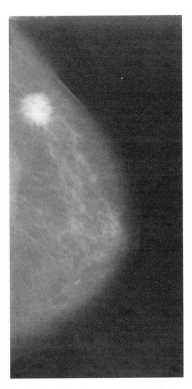

Fig. 5   Breast carcinoma: spiculated lesion.

CONDITIONS

Hormonal therapy: Used as adjuvant therapy after surgery. Tamoxifen (an anti-oestrogen with some oestrogenic effects) is the main first-line therapy for oestrogen receptor positive tumours. Others include LHRH-analogues (e.g. goserelin), progestogen and aromatase inhibitors (e.g. anastrozole, letrozole) which have recently been shown to be effective inhibition of production of oestrogen in peripheral tissues.

C: High psychological morbidity from diagnosis or physical deformity from surgery. Metastases causing bone pain, hypercalcaemia, cord compression, cerebral metastases or pulmonary complications, e.g. effusion.
From tamoxifen: Endometrial cancer, venous thrombosis.
From surgery: Wound infection, haematoma, lymphoedema, shoulder pain, sensory loss (intercostobrachial nerve is commonly sacrificed resulting in an area of numbness on the inner, upper arm), local recurrence.
From radiotherapy: Brachial plexus neuropathy (now rare), skin changes, radiation pneumonitis (a rare late complication).

P: Varies depending on stage and grade of tumour. NPI (size × 0.2 + stage + grade) predicts survival. NPI: < 3.4 15-year survival 90%, > 5.4 15-year survival 8%.

D: Tissue damage occurs by thermal, electrical or chemical injury.

A: Contact with hot object, liquids, electricity, UV light and irradiation, chemicals.

A/R: Young children and elderly at most risk and suffer ↑ mortality.

E: Common, $> 12\,000$ admissions in England and Wales annually.

H: Circumstances of burn, note time, temperature of and length of contact with agent. Consider risk of inhalation of smoke and toxic gas poisoning (carbon monoxide).

E: Look for signs of inhalational injury or airway compromise: stridor, shortness of breath, hoarse voice, soot in nose, singed nose hairs, carbonaceous sputum. Examine site, depth and distribution of burn.
Partial thickness: Subdivided into superficial and deep. Red and oedematous skin in a superficial burn, blistering and mottling in deep dermal burns; both are painful.
Full thickness: Destruction of both epidermis and dermis. Charred leathery eschar, firm and painless with loss of sensation.
Size of burn: Described as % body surface area and calculated by Wallace's 'Rule of Nines': arm or head 9%, anterior or posterior trunk 18%, leg 18%, palm area 1%, perineum 1%. Alternatively, there is the Lund–Browder Chart.

P: **Superficial partial** thickness burns involve damage to the epidermis, healing occurs within 7 days with subsequent peeling of dead skin.
Deep partial burns extend into dermis, but sweat and sebaceous glands are spared and healing occurs by epithelial regrowth over 3 weeks, usually without scarring unless infection develops.
Full thickness burns involve complete destruction of all skin layers and requires skin grafting, or healing will occur by scarring and contractures.

I: **Bloods:** $SatO_2$, ABG and carboxyhaemoglobin if an inhalational injury, FBC, U&Es and G&S or crossmatch in severe burns.
Electrical burns: Serum CK, urine myoglobin for muscle damage and ECG.

M: **Emergency: ABCs:** Secure airway, give O_2, endotracheal intubation may be necessary if inhalational injury. Assessment of size of burn, if $> 15\%$ body surface area (10% in children), IV fluids are required to prevent hypovolaemic shock. Fluid requirements can be estimated using the Muir and Barclay formula (% burn $\times \frac{1}{2}$ weight (kg)) $=$ ml fluid per time period (each 4 h from time of burn for 12 h, then each 6 h for 12 h and then 12 h); or the Parkland formula (4 ml $\times$ kg $\times$ % burn, with half the volume given over first 8 h, the other half over next 16 h). Burn should be covered with a sterile dressing, tetanus prophylaxis and analgesic given. Antibiotics are not given prophylactically (risk of resistance developing). Nutritional support in severe burns due to intensely catabolic state. Early physiotherapy to prevent development of contractures.
Surgery: Escharotomy: This is the longitudinal incision over circumferential burns to release constrictions that may compromise chest movement or limb perfusion.
Skin grafting for full thickness or deep-partial thickness once stable.

C: **Early:** Respiratory distress, hypothermia, myocardial depression, rhabdomyolysis, infection, e.g. *Streptococcus*, *Pseudomonas*, peptic ulcers (Curling's ulcer) or erosive gastritis.
Late: Hypertrophic scars and contractures.

P: Depends on the depth and extent of the burn, age and the development of complications (mortality risk approximately equal to sum of age and % burn).

CONDITIONS

Cardiac transplantation

I: Idiopathic cardiomyopathy, ischaemic heart disease, graft atherosclerosis, congenital cardiac disease, valvular cardiac disease, myocarditis.
Recipient criteria: End-stage heart disease with a life expectancy of <1 year (New York Heart Association Class III or IV).
Failure of conventional medical and surgical treatment.
No other significant systemic illness and no evidence of infection.
Emotionally stable with good compliance for immunosuppressive therapy.

A: The heart has four chambers: right and left atria and the respective ventricles. The SVC and the IVC open into the upper and lower parts of the right atrium respectively. The pulmonary artery begins at the upper part of the right ventricle passing upwards, posteriorly and to the left branching into the left and right pulmonary arteries. Four pulmonary veins open into the posterior wall of the left atrium. The aorta starts at the base of the left ventricle running anteriorly and upwards to form the ascending aorta.

I: **Pre-op:** General anaesthetic assessment.
Post-op: Should be managed in intensive care. DVT prophylaxis. Immunosuppressive therapy (e.g. cyclosporin or azathioprine) is given.

P: **Access:** A midline incision is made down the sternum and the chest wall opened with a median sternotomy. By incising and dissecting open the pericardium, the heart, coronary vessels and great vessels are exposed.
Circulatory bypass: IV systemic heparin is administered. The arterial cannula of the bypass machine is inserted in the ascending aorta for arterial outflow, while separate venous cannulae are inserted into the IVC and SVC for inflow. Systemic cooling to 26°C by the bypass machine is initiated. The aorta is crossclamped proximal to the aortic cannula while caval snares are placed across the IVC and SVC distal to the venous cannulae.
Recipient organ removal: An incision is made through both atria of the recipient's heart at mid-atrial level. The aorta is divided proximal to the aortic crossclamp while the pulmonary artery is divided just before the branching into the left and right pulmonary artery. The recipient's heart is removed in entirety.
Donor organ preparation: An incision connecting the pulmonary vein orifices is made in the left atrium of the donor heart while an incision is made in the right atrium connecting the orifices of the SVC and IVC. Careful dissection is performed to separate the aorta and pulmonary artery.
Recipient transplantation (inflow anastomosis): The donor heart is placed in the chest cavity and the left atrium is anastomosed to the remnant of the recipient's left atria with running sutures. Topical cooling with iced saline slush is applied to the donor heart externally prior to anastomosing the right atrium to the remnant of the recipient's right atria with running sutures.
Restoring circulation (and outflow anastomosis): Systemic rewarming is started while the aorta is being anastomosed with multiple interrupted sutures, after which the aortic crossclamp is removed. With the heart starting to beat, the pulmonary artery anastomosis is performed with multiple interrupted sutures. Sinus rhythm returns spontaneously or is reinstituted by cardioversion. The patient is gradually taken off the bypass circuit allowing the heart to fill and resume cardiac ejection. On satisfactory cardiac output, all cannulae are removed and protamine is administered.
Closure: Temporary pacing wires are inserted into the atrium and/or ventricles with two thoracostomy drains inserted in the pericardium and chest cavity. The sternum is closed with interrupted steel wires and the skin is closed with continuous subcuticular or interrupted sutures.

C: **Early:** Transplant rejection occurs in 70% of patients in the first 3 months. Infection affects 50% of patients within the first year.
Late: Graft atherosclerosis is found in 30–40% and 40–60% of patients at 3 years and at 5 years respectively. Transplant rejection affects less than 10% of patients per year.
Prognosis: Operative mortality rate of 3–5%. Overall 90% 1-year survival and 78% 5-year survival.

D: Narrowing of the carotid artery by atherosclerosis, a common cause of stroke.

A: Atheromatous plaque development in the region of the common carotid bifurcation.

A/R: Hypercholesterolaemia, hypertension, DM and smoking are all strong risk factors for carotid artery disease.

E: Common, affecting men more than women with increasing incidence with age.

H: May be asymptomatic.
TIAs or CVAs (responsible for 25–30%).
Amaurosis fugax (temporary unilateral vision loss – 'like a curtain coming down' caused by embolism into the ophthalmic artery, the first branch off the internal carotid artery).

E: Often normal. There may be a carotid bruit heard; however, this often does not reflect the degree of stenosis.
Signs of CVA (e.g. dysarthria, dysphasia, weakness in limbs).
Signs of systemic vascular disease.

P: The carotid artery bifurcation is an area of the vascular tree where atherosclerosis is common. In combination with systemic risk factors, local haemodynamics, including low shear stress and ↑ turbulence affecting the outer walls opposite the flow divider predispose to atheroma development, luminal narrowing and risk of plaque rupture, thrombosis or embolism (see Fig. 6).

I: **Duplex Doppler ultrasound:** Non-invasive imaging to assess degree of stenosis.
Angiography: Invasive procedure carrying a risk of precipitating a stroke (1% CVA, 4% TIA), but allows more accurate assessment of stenosis severity.
MRA: Also non-invasive.

M: **Medical:** For asymptomatic or < 70% internal carotid artery stenosis; at present, recommended treatment is medical, i.e. low-dose aspirin, stopping smoking and treatment of other risk factors, hypercholesterolaemia, hypertension and diabetes.
Surgical: For symptomatic (within last 6 months) internal carotid artery stenosis > 70–99% or if the plaque is ulcerated, carotid endarterectomy has been shown to reduce risk of stroke (ECST and NASCET). Trials are underway to ascertain if asymptomatic stenosis should be surgically treated and also comparing local and general anaesthesia.
Angioplasty +/− stenting: The CAVATAS trial shows endovascular treatment has similar major risks and effectiveness at preventing stroke over 3 years but a greater rate of re-stenosis and immediate post-op stroke. The CREST and ICSS trial are underway, comparing endarterectomy and endovascular stenting.

C: **Complications of disease:** Cerebrovascular attacks.
Complications from surgery: Cardiac ischaemia or infarction (3%), cranial nerve injury (2–7%, usually recurrent laryngeal nerve or hypoglossal nerves), haematoma with or without airway compromise, hypertension, hypotension, peri-operative stroke (1–5%). The peri-operative mortality rate is 0.5–1.8%.

P: For carotid artery stenosis of > 70%, annual stroke rate is 10–20%. If untreated, asymptomatic stenosis of 50% has an annual stroke risk of 1%.
If surgically corrected: Results in a six- to eightfold reduction in risk of stroke compared to best medical therapy alone in patients with severe stenosis.

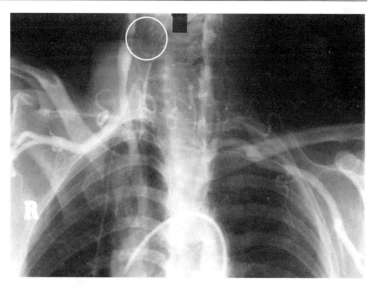

Fig. 6 Arteriogram showing atheromatous carotid arteries and right carotid stenosis.

D: A tumour arising from chemoreceptor cells at the carotid bifurcation, also known as a chemodectoma.

A: Unknown, 10% are familial with autosomal dominant inheritance. In these cases, tumours are more likely to be bilateral and multiple (30%).

A/R: There is an ↑ incidence in those who live at high altitudes for long periods.

E: Rare. Any age may present, most commonly 50–70 years, now women > men.

H: Most commonly presents as a slowly growing lump in the neck. Pressure on nearby cranial nerves may give rise to symptoms such as dysphagia, choking or hoarseness.

E: Neck lump in the region of the carotid triangle of the neck with transmitted pulsation. There may be evidence of cranial nerve VII, IX, X, XI paresis or palsy.

P: Carotid body tumour is a form of paraganglioma, which includes vagal body tumours, glomus jugulare tumours and pheochromocytomas.
Micro: Vascular tumour with epithelioid 'chief cells' arranged in clusters within a fibrous stroma. The cells are usually nonsecretory (although have the potential to secrete adrenaline or noradrenaline).
Macro: The margins are well defined and most are benign with < 20% undergoing local invasion or metastases to lymph nodes or more commonly, bone. In 10% of cases, tumours will be bilateral or multiple.

I: **USG, duplex scanning:** Will show the relationship with the carotid bifurcation, angiography confirms the characteristic splaying of the internal and external carotid arteries and the tumour 'blush in wine glass' appearance.
CT or MRI scan: Used to determine the extent of the tumour.
Direct and indirect pharyngoscopy and laryngoscopy: May be performed to assess cranial nerve involvement or pharyngeal invasion.
FNA: Cytology can be used in diagnosis.

M: **Conservative approach:** May be taken if the patient is frail and elderly.
Surgery: As they are very vascular, pre-op embolisation of large tumours is carried out and several units of blood should be crossmatched. Surgical excision of the tumour: an incision is made along the anterior border of sternocleidomastoid and the carotid artery bifurcation exposed. The external carotid artery is often clamped or isolated by placement of a shunt from the common carotid into the internal carotid artery to reduce the blood flow to the tumour. Transcranial Doppler can be used to monitor distal flow. If the tumour is significantly adherent or invading an artery wall, it may be necessary to excise an arterial segment replacing it with a length of saphenous vein. Craniofacial surgeons are involved if the tumour extends high into the neck.
Radiotherapy: To prevent local recurrence when local invasion has occurred and to treat metastatic disease.

C: **Tumour:** Local invasion causing cranial nerve palsies, distal metastases.
Surgery: 10–20% experience neurological deficits (mandibular branch of VII, IX, X, especially the recurrent laryngeal nerves, XII) resulting in possible respiratory or swallowing difficulties, but most recover. There is also a small risk of stroke (< 3%).

P: Characteristically slow growing; however, if untreated, 75% develop symptoms and 30% die from invasion and metastases. Most patients are cured by surgery.

CONDITIONS

Carotid endarterectomy

I: TIAs or strokes in the previous 6 months in the distribution of the diseased carotid artery with stenosis of 70–99% ipsilateral or > 50% bilaterally, ulcerated plaques (ECST and NASCET).

A: The principal arterial supply of the head and neck are the two common carotids. The common carotid arteries differ in length and in their mode of origin. The right begins at the bifurcation of the innominate artery behind the sternoclavicular joint and is confined to the neck. The left springs from the highest part of the arch of the aorta to the left of, and on a plane posterior to, the innominate artery, and therefore consists of a thoracic and a cervical portion. They ascend in the neck dividing into two branches:

(1) the external carotid supplies the exterior of the skull, the face and the greater part of the neck. The first branch after the carotid bifurcation is the superior thyroid artery.

(2) the internal carotid supplies virtually everything within the cranium and orbit.

I: **Pre-op:** Carotid duplex is first-line investigation to quantify extent of stenosis. Carotid angiogram may be necessary to assess the extent of the disease and the superior extent of the stenosis. Concomitant coronary artery disease is common, so an echocardiogram, a coronary angiogram, and serum cholesterol levels may be necessary. Baseline ECG. CT head (for evidence of previous CVAs).

Post-op: Frequent neurologic assessment should be carried out as well as haemodynamic and ECG monitoring. Observe the patient for a haematoma that may compromise the airway. Antiplatelet therapy is necessary.

Follow-up care: Re-evaluation should be done 2 weeks post-op for complications. Carotid duplex is performed after 6 months and then annually.

P: **Anaesthesia:** Local anaesthesia has the advantage of allowing direct evaluation of the patient's neurological status without sophisticated monitoring. This enables the surgeon to operate on the majority of patients without the need for a shunt. General anaesthesia has the advantage of improved airway control and patient comfort during prolonged operations. However, it does require the use of shunts, and selective shunting requires the use of EEG, stump pressures, transcranial Doppler and/or some other form of cerebral monitoring.

Incision: An incision should be made along the anterior border of the sternocleidomastoid muscle. An oblique incision is usually made in the skinfold over the carotid bifurcation.

Dissecting the common and internal carotid: Short tapes are used to isolate the proximal common carotid and distal internal carotid. The common and internal carotid is carefully dissected taking care not to jar the artery and trigger embolism.

Dissecting the external carotid: The external carotid is dissected and a short tape is looped around it as well. The carotid body may be accidentally stimulated triggering BP instability.

Removal of plaque: Heparin can be started once all vessels are controlled. A shunt may be used at this point. Arteriotomy is performed distal to the site of the stenosis. The plaque is removed distal to proximal in one piece with gentle traction.

Closure: The arteriotomy is closed with full thickness sutures while simultaneously removing the shunt. Before final closure, artery may be irrigated with heparinised saline. The arteriotomy can be closed directly or with a prosthetic or vein patch. The technical result should be verified by completion duplex ultrasound.

C: Cardiac ischaemia, cranial nerve injury (2–7%, usually recurrent laryngeal nerve or hypoglossal nerves), haematoma with or without airway compromise, hypertension, hypotension, peri-operative stroke (1–5%). The peri-operative mortality rate is 0.5–1.8%.

D: Opacification of the lens of the eye.

A: Majority of cases are idiopathic age-related ('senile cataracts'). Numerous secondary causes including:
Local: Previous eye trauma, uveitis, intraocular tumours.
Systemic: DM, metabolic disorders (galactosaemia, hypocalcaemia, Wilson's disease), skin disease (atopic dermatitis, scleroderma), drugs (steroids), X-ray and UV radiation, myotonic dystrophy, genetic syndromes (Down's).
Congenital: Congenital rubella syndrome.

A/R: Nil.

E: Major cause of treatable blindness worldwide.

H: Gradual onset painless loss of vision.
Glare from bright light, vision may worsen in bright light (especially with central lens opacity).
Some may experience monocular diplopia and see haloes around lights.
Some may notice that they can read without glasses (nuclear sclerotic cataract may ↑ lens-converging power).
In infants, there may be amblyopia or nystagmus.

E: Loss of red reflex and hazy lens appearance.
Reduced visual acuity.

P: **(Seen with slit-lamp microscope):** In the early stages, there is compression of lens fibre in the central portion of the lens (nuclear sclerosis), with gradual change of the crystalline lens nucleus from translucent to brown or gray. There may be areas of granular opacities (e.g. in posterior subcapsular subtype).

I: Unnecessary unless occuring at an early age or in background of systemic disease.

M: Congenital cataracts must be treated urgently to avoid amblyopia.
The decision for surgery depends on the effect of the cataracts on the patient's vision and life.
Surgical: Phacoemulsification (using ultrasound probe) followed by aspiration of lens material and insertion of intraocular lens implant is curative. Specific complications include posterior capsule opacification, vitreous humour loss, and endophthalmitis. Usually done as day surgery. Post-op care should include steroid drops (for inflammation), antibiotic drops (infection prophylaxis), avoidance of strenuous exercise and ocular trauma.

C: None, other than reduced quality of life from reduced visual acuity.

P: Good with treatment for age-related cataracts.

PROCEDURES

I: Administration of toxic drugs, parenteral nutrition or hyperosmotic agents. Central venous pressure monitoring.

Venous access where peripheral venous access is difficult, e.g. in IV drug abusers or where repeated access is required, e.g. haemodialysis or haemofiltration.

Placement of cardiac pacing wires.

Vascular access during interventional radiological procedures, e.g. angiography, transjugular intrahepatic portosystemic shunt placement, organ biopsy or selective venous sampling.

A: **Internal jugular:** The internal jugular vein starts at the jugular foramen and runs down the neck on the carotid sheath and meets the subclavian behind the medial end of the clavicle. The common carotid artery lies medially; the subclavian artery, thyrocervical trunk, vertebral vein, cervical plexus, phrenic nerve, scalenus medius and anterior muscles sit posteriorly while anteriolaterally is the sternocleidomastoid muscle.

Subclavian: The subclavian vein begins at the outer border of the first rib and lies posterior to the clavicle and subclavius muscle, anterior to scalenus anterior muscle and phrenic nerve and superior to the first rib. It joins the internal jugular vein at the medial border of the scalenus anterior muscle to form the brachiocephalic vein.

Femoral: The femoral vein originates at the saphenous opening in the thigh and accompanies the femoral artery ending at the inguinal ligament, where it becomes the external iliac vein. In the femoral triangle, the femoral vein lies medial to the artery, between the artery and the femoral canal. The femoral nerve lies lateral to the artery.

I: **Pre-procedure:** It is wise to check the patient's clotting status before starting the procedure. The procedure should be explained to the patient and consent gained if possible. A continuous cardiac monitor is also useful. All three lumens of the central venous catheter should be flushed with saline before starting.

Post-procedure: It is vital to perform a CXR to confirm the position of internal jugular and subclavian CVP lines and to exclude any complications such as pneumothorax. The catheter should lie above the junction of the SVC and the right atrium.

P: Guidelines suggest that this procedure should be carried out more safely with handheld ultrasound guidance (if available) to help identify the vein and avoid the artery.

Position: 15° head down, to distend the upper body veins, with head turned away.

Internal jugular venepuncture:

(1) The skin is sterilised and draped exposing an area in the center of the triangle formed by the two heads of sternocleidomastoid and the clavicle. The carotid artery is palpated and held in place medially at the level of the cricoid cartilage. This area is marked and infiltrated with 1% lignocaine.

(2) Using a needle and syringe, the skin over the marked area is punctured. The direction of the advance is parallel to the sagittal plane, in the caudal direction and 30° posteriorly ('aiming for the nipple on the same side'). The needle is advanced while aspirating until there is a flush of blood in the syringe. The needle is then advanced a further 2 mm. If the vein is not encountered, the needle is withdrawn to skin level and redirected.

Subclavian venepuncture:

(1) The skin is sterilised and draped exposing an area 1 cm below and lateral to the midclavicular point. This area is marked and infiltrated with 1% lignocaine.

(2) Using a needle and syringe, the skin over the marked point is punctured with the needle. The direction of the advance is horizontal and medial, aiming to go behind the clavicle towards the suprasternal notch. If the clavicle is hit, the needle is withdrawn and angled slightly deeper. The needle is advanced while aspirating until there is a flush of blood in the syringe. The needle is then advanced a further 2 mm.

Femoral venepuncture:

(1) The skin is sterilised and draped exposing an area inferior to the ilio-inguinal ligament and about 1 cm medial to the femoral pulse. The femoral artery is palpated and held in place laterally. This area is marked and infiltrated with 1% lignocaine.

(2) Using a needle and syringe, the skin over the marked point is punctured with the needle. The direction of the advance is medial aiming towards the head, at about 20–30° angle to the skin plane. The needle is advanced while aspirating until there is a flush of blood in the syringe. The needle is then advanced a further 2 mm.

Confirmation of vein: Leaving the needle in place, the syringe is removed. The blood flow from the needle should not be pulsatile. If the blood flow is pulsatile or if the blood is arterial in appearance, the needle is removed and firm pressure is placed over the site until there is haemostasis. Return to the first step.

Guide-wire insertion: A guide wire is passed through the needle and should advance without resistance. If not, reattach the syringe, check for free flow blood and adjust as necessary. The needle is removed once the guide wire is in place. The guide wire must always be held throughout the procedure to ensure that it is not lost into the circulation.

Dilator: The skin entry point is enlarged with a scalpel and a dilator is passed over the guide wire and then removed.

Central venous catheter insertion: The catheter is passed over the guide wire. The guide wire is removed when the catheter is in place. Free flow of blood from the catheter is confirmed before flushing the catheter with saline.

Securing the catheter: The catheter is sutured in position, a sterile dressing applied and the tubing taped in place.

C: Pneumothorax, haemothorax (especially by subclavian route), air embolism, arterial puncture, skin or line infection (especially by femoral route). Cardiac arrhythmias (e.g. ventricular or atrial ectopics) may be induced if the guide wire is inserted too far.

Cholangiocarcinoma

D: Primary adenocarcinoma of the biliary tree.

A: Aetiology of the majority of cholangiocarcinomas are unknown.

A/R: Known associations are ulcerative colitis and PSC, choledochal cysts, Caroli's disease and parasitic infections of the biliary tract (e.g. *Clonorchis sinensis* liver flukes).

E: Rare, accounting for ~0.2–0.3% of all cancers. Outnumbered by gallbladder and pancreatic carcinoma. Slightly more common in males. More common in developing world due to parasitic infestations.

H: Obstructive jaundice (yellow skin and sclera, pale stools, dark urine, pruritus). Abdominal fullness or pain.
Symptoms of malignancy: Weight loss, malaise.

E: Jaundice. Palpable gallbladder (Courvoisier's law states that, in the presence of jaundice, an enlarged gallbladder is unlikely to be due to gallstones; i.e. carcinoma of the pancreas or the lower biliary tree is more likely).
Epigastric or right upper quadrant mass.
There may be hepatomegaly.

P: **Micro:** Adenocarcinoma arising from biliary tract, papillary, nodular or sclerosing types. Usually moderately differentiated and slow-growing.
Macro: Described according to location into hilar, mid-duct, distal and diffuse.
Bismuth classification of hilar tumours into types I to V based on their location in relation to the confluence of hepatic ducts. Klatskin tumours are cholangiocarcinomas arising at the confluence of the left and right hepatic ducts.
Staging: TNM staging.

I: **Bloods:** FBC, U&Es, LFT (bilirubin, alkphos and γ-GT raised), clotting, tumour markers (CA19-9 raised in cholangiocarcinomas and pancreatic carcinomas).
Endoscopy: ERCP enables bile cytology, tumour biopsy if accessible and interventions to relieve obstructive jaundice.
Radiology: Ultrasound: Variable sensitivity but will show biliary duct dilation.
CT, MRI or MRCP, bone scan: To stage tumour and visualise any regional spread.
Arteriogram (invasive or MR): Important when considering surgery to show any involvement of surrounding vascular structures.

M: **Medical:** Palliative measures in unresectable tumours. Endoscopic (or percutaneous) insertion of stents (plastic or metal) or internal–external drains.
Chemo/Radiotherapy: Intracavity or brachytherapy can be quite effective in reducing tumour size. Chemotherapy response rates are relatively poor at present.
Surgical: <15% are resectable. Proximal tumours are resected along with associated liver lobe. Distal tumours can be treated with Whipple's procedure (proximal pancreaticoduodenectomy with choledocho- or hepaticojejunostomy, i.e. resection of the pancreatic head, together with the distal stomach, duodenum, upper jejunum, and the gallbladder, and reconstruction by anastomosis of the proximal biliary tree to the jejunum).

C: Metastases (lymphatic or local hepatic spread are usual routes), obstructive jaundice, cholangitis.

P: Poor. Most patients die within 1 year if unresected. 5-year survival rate of resected tumours is about 40%.

I: Symptomatic cholelithiasis, now one of the most commonly performed operations. Can be carried out in the acute setting (within 72 h of onset of acute cholecystitis); however, there is ↑ complication rate, and operation is best delayed a few weeks until inflammation has settled.

A: The gallbladder lies on the inferior surface of the liver. It is divided into fundus, body, infundibulum and neck that may develop a Hartmann's pouch. The cystic duct connects the gallbladder to the junction of the common hepatic duct and bile duct and the musosa forms folds known as the spiral valve of Heister. Anatomic variants are common (e.g. the cystic duct draining into the right hepatic duct).

Vascular supply: From the cystic artery, a branch of the right hepatic artery. This lies in Calot's triangle, made up by the lower edge of the liver, common hepatic duct medially and the cystic duct inferiorly. Small vessels and ducts (of Luschka) may run directly between the liver and the gallbladder. An important vascular anomaly is an aberrant right hepatic artery that comes from the superior mesenteric artery, and runs in a groove between the common hepatic duct and portal vein at the medial border of Calot's triangle.

I: **Pre-op:** Patients would have had an abdominal ultrasound to diagnose gallstones. FBC, U&Es, LFT, clotting and G&S are baseline blood tests.
Post-op: DVT prophylaxis. Patients may often be discharged the next day.

P: Patients should have an empty bladder, an NG tube is placed if the stomach is distended, antibiotic prophyaxis is given.

Laparoscope insertion: The primary trocar is introduced using an open or closed technique; the former is a safer way whereby a small incision (usually subumbilical) is made with dissection and opening of the peritoneal cavity under direct vision. A pneumoperitoneum is created by insufflation of CO_2. After inspection, three further ports are introduced under direct vision (11 mm port in epigastrium, two 5.5 mm ports along the right costal margin).

Cholecystectomy: The infundibulum of the gallbladder is picked up with grasping forceps via the right port and pulled to the right. Calot's triangle is dissected by forceps and diathermy to identify the cystic duct and cystic artery (vigilance is important for anatomical variation in this area). The cystic duct is clipped near the gallbladder and an intraoperative cholangiogram can be performed to identify stones in the common bile duct if required. The cystic artery and duct are clipped proximally and distally, then divided between the clips.

Mobilisation of gallbladder: The gallbladder is mobilised and inspected to ensure that there are no accessory hepatic ducts. The gallbladder is then pulled to the right and slightly cranially and dissected away from the undersurface of the liver. Any bleeding vessels are treated with electrocauterisation. Spilled gallstones should be retrieved if possible.

Closure: The gallbladder is placed in a plastic sac and extracted via a port. The right upper quadrant is thoroughly irrigated and the fluid then suctioned from the subphrenic space. The ports are removed and the wounds are closed.

C: **Early:** Infection, haemorrhage, bile leak, injury to common bile duct or other biliary ducts. If complications (e.g. difficulty in identifying anatomy, haemorrhage, damage to another structure) develop, conversion to open cholecystectomy should be performed.
Late: Postcholecystectomy syndrome (persistant dyspeptic symptoms), port-site hernias.

Cholecystectomy, Open

I: **Open:** (1) Suspected gallbladder cancer
(2) Liver cirrhosis with portal hypertension
Conversion from laparoscopic:
(1) Inability to identify anatomy
(2) Multiple adhesions
(3) Intraoperative metabolic acidosis

A: The gallbladder lies on the undersurface of the liver, bound to it by the peritoneum. It is divided into a fundus, body, infundibulum and neck that may develop a Hartmann's pouch. The cystic duct connects the gallbladder to the junction of the common hepatic duct and bile duct and the musosa forms folds, known as the spiral valve of Heister. Anatomic variants are common, e.g. the cystic duct draining into the right hepatic duct.
Vascular supply: From the cystic artery, a branch of the right hepatic artery. This lies in Calot's triangle, made up by the lower edge of the liver, common hepatic duct medially and the cystic duct inferiorly. Small vessels and ducts (of Luschka) may run directly between the liver and the gallbladder. An important vascular anomaly is an aberrant right hepatic artery that comes from the superior mesenteric artery, and runs in a groove between the common hepatic duct and portal vein at the medial border of Calot's triangle.

I: **Pre-op:** Patients have had imaging to identify relevant pathology, e.g. USS, CT or MRI. FBC, U&Es, LFT, clotting studies and G&S are minimal baseline blood tests.
Post-op: DVT prophylaxis.

P: **Access:** A transverse subcostal (for good cosmetic result) or a midline (for speed and good access) incision is made.
Mobilisation of gallbladder: The gallbladder is exposed and the peritoneum overlying the cystic duct and artery dissected.
Ligation of cystic vessels: The cystic artery is identified, dissected free, clamped, ligated and divided. The cystic duct is identified, dissected free and ligated to prevent the passage of stones from the gallbladder into the common bile duct.
Cholecystectomy: The gallbladder is dissected free from the liver with dissection continued to expose the junction of the cystic duct and the common bile duct (intraoperative cholangiography can now be performed via a small incision in the cystic duct and cannulation). The cystic duct is ligated proximally and distally, and then divided. The gallbladder is removed from the surgical field.
Closure: The wound is closed in three layers: the posterior rectus sheath and the peritoneum are closed with a continuous suture, the anterior rectus sheath is closed with a separate continuous suture and the skin is closed with a continuous subcuticular suture, interrupted sutures or with staples. Drainage is not usually required.

C: Infection, haemorrhage, injury to common bile duct or other biliary ducts.

I: **Elective:** Most commonly performed in infants or young boys for religious or cultural reasons. Recurrent balanoposthitis (infection of the foreskin and penis), phimosis, paraphimosis, balanitis xerotica obliterans (lichen sclerosus of the foreskin), penile carcinoma.
Contraindications: Hypospadias, chordee and buried penis.
Emergency: Presentation with severely inflamed/infected foreskin or penis; in these cases a dorsal slit of the phimotic foreskin is safer, as there is a risk of exacerbating infection and poor cosmesis. A formal circumcision is performed once infection and swelling have settled down.

A: The foreskin covers and protects the glans and external urethral meatus. Separation from the glans occurs gradually in young boys and is complete in 90% by age 5 years. Consists of stratified squamous epithelium with underlying lamina propria and dartos muscle layers.
Vascular supply: Dorsal artery from the internal pudendal artery and superficial branches of the external pudendal arteries anastomose to supply the penile skin. Venous drainage is via the superficial dorsal vein that drains into the superficial external pudendal vein.
Nerve supply: Innervation is by the dorsal nerve of the penis (a branch of the pudendal nerve) and branches of the perineal nerves from S2, S3 and S4.

I: If patient is healthy, no particular pre-op investigations are necessary.

P: Can be performed as a day procedure under general anaesthesia +/− caudal or local penile block.
Procedure: Most common technique involves making a dorsal slit and then dissecting and excising the foreskin with careful haemostasis. Suture of the penile skin to mucosa at the corona is carried out using interrupted absorbable sutures. A gauze dressing is placed around the wound to prevent adherence to undergarments. The foreskin is routinely sent for histological examination.
Forceps-guided circumcision (alternative method): The foreskin is pulled forward in front of the glans, a forceps clamped across it and excised with a scalpel. The cut edges of the inner and outer skin are then sutured.

C: **Early:** Haemorrhage (1–2%), penile injury (e.g. diathermy burns), urinary retention, infection.
Late: Meatal stenosis or ulcer, urethral fistula, recurrent phimosis due to inadequate circumcision, chordee due to excessive skin removal.

P: Usually a straightforward procedure but haemorrhage can be problematic.

Colonic polyps

CONDITIONS

D: A growth from the bowel wall that projects into the colonic lumen.

A: A common occurrence. Classified into non-neoplastic and neoplastic polyps, most of which are benign proliferations of mucosa and submucosa (adenomas), but clinically significant due to malignant potential (see Colorectal carcinoma).

A/R: Multiple colonic polyps occur in some syndromes.

Disorder	Features
Peutz–Jeghers syndrome	Diffuse GI polyposis with mucocutaneous pigmentation of lips and gums. Benign.
Familial polyposis coli	Multiple stomach, small and large bowel adenomas. Autosomal dominant APC gene. Pre-malignant.
Gardner's syndrome	Osteomas, soft tissue tumours, sebaceous cysts, congenital hypertrophy of RPE and multiple colonic adenomas. Pre-malignant.
Turcot's syndrome	Glioblastomas or medulloblastomas, with multiple colonic adenomas. Pre-malignant.
Cronkhite–Canada's syndrome	Alopecia, nail atrophy, pigmentation, watery diarrhoea, multiple colonic adenomas. Pre-malignant.

E: Common. Prevalence is $> 50\%$ in those > 60 years.

H: Usually asymptomatic.
May cause a change in bowel habit, mucoid diarrhoea, PR bleeding or symptoms of anaemia.

E: Usually no findings on examination.
May be palpable on PR examination if low in rectum.
Associated features of multiple polyposis syndromes.

P: **Macro:** May be sessile or pedunculated. Size ranges from mm to cm in diameter.
Micro: Non-neoplastic polyps include metaplastic (hyperplastic), inflammatory and hamartomatous polyps. Neoplastic polyps are adenomas, either tubular, tubulovillous or villous, the latter with the greater tendency to malignancy.

I: **Bloods:** FBC (anaemia).
Stool: Occult or frank blood in stool.
Endoscopy: Colonoscopy is gold standard investigation. For multiple polyposis syndromes, an upper GI endoscopy is necessary to look for upper GI polyps. Polyps removed need to be histologically examined to exclude malignant change.

M: **Endoscopy:** Colonoscopic polypectomy for small isolated polyps.
Surgical: Large polyps may have to be surgically resected. In multiple polyposis syndromes (particularly familial polyposis coli), early subtotal colectomy is recommended to reduce risk of malignancy.
Follow-up: Patients should be followed up with colonoscopy every 2–4 years. Genetic screening of relatives may be necessary in multiple polyposis syndromes.

C: Malignant change with highest risk in villous adenomas and in multiple polyposis syndromes. Risk of bowel obstruction.

P: Good if detected and treated before any malignant change.

D: Malignant adenocarcinoma of the large bowel.

A: Environmental and genetic factors have been implicated. A sequence from epithelial dysplasia leading to adenoma and then carcinoma is thought to occur involving accumulation of genetic changes in oncogenes, (e.g. APC, K-ras) and tumour suppressor genes (e.g. p53, DCC).

A/R: Western diet (high intake of red meat, alcohol, fat, sugar and reduced vege-table and fibre intake), presence of colorectal polyps, previous colorectal cancer, family history, IBD (particularly longstanding ulcerative colitis). Familial syndromes associated with ↑ risk (see Colonic polyps).

E: Second most common cause of cancer death in the West. 20 000 deaths per year in the UK. Average age at diagnosis 60–65 years. Rectal carcinomas male > female, colon carcinomas female > male.

H: Symptoms will depend on the location of the tumour.
Left-sided colon and rectum: Change in bowel habit, rectal bleeding or blood/mucus mixed in with stools. Rectal masses may also present as tenesmus (sensation of incomplete emptying after defecation).
Right-sided colon: Later presentation, with symptoms of anaemia, weight loss and nonspecific malaise or more rarely, lower abdominal pain.
Up to 20% of tumours will present as an emergency with pain and distension due to LBO, haemorrhage or peritonitis due to perforation.

E: Anaemia may be the only sign, particularly in right-sided lesions, abdominal mass, with metastatic disease, hepatomegaly, 'shifting dullness' of ascites. Low-lying rectal tumours may be palpable on rectal examination.

P: **Macro:** 60% rectum and sigmoid colon, 30% in the ascending colon and the remainder in the descending and transverse colon. Distal colon tumours tend to form an annular encircling ring around the bowel wall, causing 'apple core' constrictions (see Fig. 7a); proximal colon tumours tend to form polypoid, exophytic masses.
Micro: Neoplastic change with deranged adenomatous or anaplastic cells and varying degrees of bowel wall penetration. Staging systems include Dukes' (see below) and the TNM system.

I: **Bloods:** FBC (for anaemia), LFT, tumour markers (CEA to monitor treatment response or disease recurrence).
Stool: Occult or frank blood in stool (can be used as a screening test).
Endoscopy: Sigmoidoscopy, colonoscopy. Allows visualisation and biopsy. Polypectomy can also be done if isolated small carcinoma in situ.
Barium contrast studies: 'Apple core' stricture on barium enema.
Contrast CT scan: For staging.
Other staging investigations include CXR, MRI, endorectal ultrasound.

M: **Surgery:** This is the only curative treatment. Operation depends on circum-stance (see the various Colorectal resections and Fig. 7b).

Caecum	Right hemicolectomy
High rectum	Anterior resection
Low rectum	Abdominoperineal resection and end colostomy formation
Emergency	Hartmann's procedure (proximal colostomy, resection of tumour and closure of rectal stump)

CONDITIONS

Survival in rectal tumours is improved if total mesorectal excision (removal of surrounding fascia). Hepatic metastases may be cured by resection.

Radiotherapy: May be given in a neoadjuvant setting to downstage rectal tumours prior to resection or as adjuvant therapy to reduce risk of local recurrence.

Chemotherapy: Used as adjuvant therapy in Dukes' C or sometimes B. 5-fluorouracil is a commonly used drug, others are being assessed in clinical trials.

C: Bowel obstruction or perforation, fistula formation, recurrence, metastatic disease.

P: Varies depending on Dukes' staging.

Dukes	Extent of spread	5-yr survival (%)
A	Confined to bowel wall	80–90
B	Breached serosa but no lymph nodes	60
C	Breached serosa with lymph nodes	30
D	Distant metastases (usually liver)	< 5

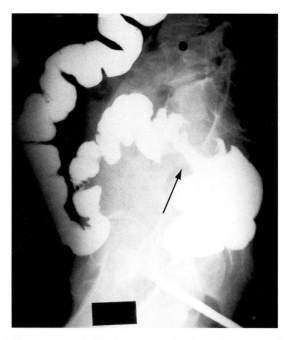

Fig. 7a Barium enema study showing stenosing (apple core) carcinoma of the colon.

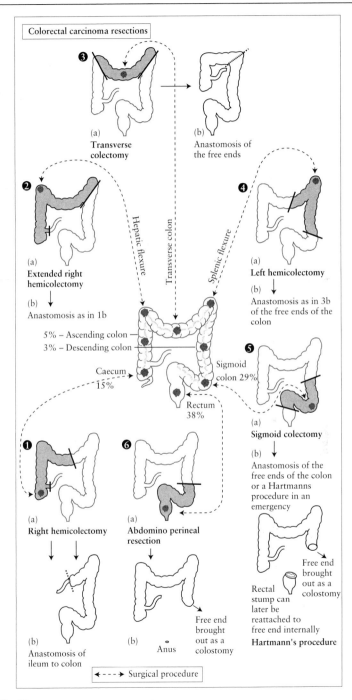

Colorectal carcinoma resections

❸ (a) Transverse colectomy

(b) Anastomosis of the free ends

❷ (a) Extended right hemicolectomy

(b) ↓ Anastomosis as in 1b

Hepatic flexure
Transverse colon
Splenic flexure

5% – Ascending colon
3% – Descending colon

Caecum 15%

Sigmoid colon 29%

Rectum 38%

❹ (a) Left hemicolectomy

(b) ↓ Anastomosis as in 3b of the free ends of the colon

❺ (a) Sigmoid colectomy

(b) ↓ Anastomosis of the free ends of the colon or a Hartmanns procedure in an emergency

Free end brought out as a colostomy

Rectal stump can later be reattached to free end internally

Hartmann's procedure

❶ (a) Right hemicolectomy ↓   ↓

(b) Anastomosis of ileum to colon

❻ (a) Abdomino perineal resection ↓

(b) Anus

Free end brought out as a colostomy

◀---▶ Surgical procedure

Fig. 7b

CONDITIONS

Colorectal resection, Abdomino-perineal

I: **Elective:** Tumours of the lower rectum and anus.

A: The rectum begins at the level of the third sacral vertebra, passes downward, lying in the sacrococcygeal curve, and extends anterior to the tip of the coccyx. It then bends sharply backward into the anal canal. The rectum is about 12 cm long, and is surrounded by a dense tube of fascia derived from the endopelvic fascia, but fused behind with the fascia covering the sacrum and coccyx.

Vascular: The inferior mesenteric artery supplies the upper rectum via the superior rectal artery. The middle rectal artery supplies the lower rectum and derives from the internal iliac artery. Both arteries form an anastomosis. The rectal venous plexus drains into the superior, middle and inferior rectal vessels. The rectal venous plexus is a site of portacaval connection.

Lymphatics: Drainage follows the inferior mesenteric artery to para-aortic nodes.

I: **CT-scan:** For planning and assessing suitability for an abdominoperineal excision and to exclude metastatic disease.

Pre-op: Nil by mouth, bowel preparation, urinary catheterisation.

Post-op: NG tube, IV fluids, monitor FBC and electrolytes.

P: Patient is positioned with legs in the lithotomy position with slight head-down tilt and legs parted. The anal opening is sutured shut.

Incision: Lower midline incision.

Mobilising the sigmoid: See Anterior resection.

Mobilising the rectum: See Anterior resection.

Mobilising the anus: Perianal surgery needs to be treated as nonsterile, and is usually performed by another surgeon. An elliptical incision is made around the sutured anal opening, extending posteriorly to the coccyx and associated fascial plane. The levator ani is divided posterior to anterior around the anus. The incision is then deepened until connection is made with the abdominal side of the surgery. The superficial transverse muscles are divided anteriorly. The anus and rectum are then removed from the perineal side.

Resection: The bowel is divided between clamps and a colostomy is fashioned in the LIF (see Fig. 7b).

Closure: A pelvic drain should be left in situ. The abdominal wall is closed with nylon sutures while the perineal surface is closed with subcuticular sutures.

C: Necrosis of the stoma or perineal wound, wound infection, persistent ileus, ischaemic bowel, peritonitis, tumour recurrence.

I: **Elective:** Rectal tumours (> 2 cm from dentate line), diverticular disease.

A: The rectum begins at the level of the third sacral vertebra, passes downward, lying in the sacrococcygeal curve, and extends anterior to the tip of the coccyx. It then bends sharply backward into the anal canal. The rectum is about 12 cm long, and is surrounded by a dense tube of fascia derived from the endopelvic fascia, but fused behind with the fascia covering the sacrum and coccyx. The anterior fascia is called Denonvillier's fascia.
Vascular: The inferior mesenteric artery supplies the upper rectum via the superior rectal artery. The middle rectal artery supplies the lower rectum and derives from the internal iliac artery. These arteries anastomose with each other. The rectal venous plexus drains into the superior, middle and inferior rectal vessels that run on the anterolateral surface of the rectal wall. The rectal venous plexus is a site of portacaval connection.
Lymphatics: Drainage follows the inferior mesenteric artery to para-aortic nodes.

I: **CT scan:** For planning and assessing suitability for anterior resection and to exclude metastatic disease. Pre-op radiotherapy may improve the staging of the disease.
Pre-op: Nil by mouth, bowel preparation, FBC, U&Es, clotting and crossmatch, general anaesthetic assessment and appropriate investigations.
Post-op: NG tube, IV fluids, close monitoring of FBC, electrolytes and urine output. DVT prophylaxis.

P: Patient is positioned in the lithotomy position with slight head-down tilt.
Incision: Lower or extended midline incision.
Mobilising the colon: Initial assessment of the size and extent of the tumour is made. The sigmoid mesentery may be dissected, identifing and ligating branches of the inferior mesenteric artery, carefully identifying the ureter and gonadal vessels in the process.
Mobilising the rectum: The posterior dissection plane of the rectum is created by blunt finger dissection of the avascular presacral fascia, carefully avoiding the sacral plexus. The anterior dissection plane is created by blunt dissection and countertraction of Denonvillier's fascia, separating the rectum from the bladder, prostate (in males), uterus and vagina (in females). In low anterior resections, the lateral ligaments are also dissected.
Resection: Adequate clearance of at least 2 cm is needed proximal and distal to the tumour. Clamps are placed at the distal and proximal resection sites. The lower rectum and anus are washed via proctoscope with antiseptic solution. The bowel is then divided between the proximal and distal clamps.
Anastomosis: Most surgeons use a stapling gun. The gun is inserted PR by an assistant and the distal rectum is sutured around the stapler with a purse string. Meanwhile, the proximal bowel end is sutured around the receiving end of the stapler gun (the anvil). The stapler is now closed, which results in a ring of bowel being excised and the two ends being stapled together. The 'doughnut' tissue excised is examined to ensure a complete ring. The anastomosis can be checked by submerging underwater and inflating air into the anus from a proctoscope to look for bubbles.
Closure: A pelvic drain is usually left in situ. The abdominal wall is closed with non-absorbable sutures. Skin closure is completed with sutures or clips. Defunctioning stomas may be fashioned.

C: **Specific:** Anastomotic leak resulting in abscess formation or peritonitis, persistent ileus, ischaemic bowel, tumour recurrence at anal margin. Post-op anorectal function may be impaired for up to 18 months post procedure.

I: Elective: Tumours of the splenic flexure, descending colon and proximal sigmoid colon are the commonest indications. Severe diverticular disease.
Emergency: Occasionally indicated for obstruction, perforation or ischaemia.

A: The descending colon passes downward through the left hypochondrium and lumbar regions along the lateral border of the left kidney. The peritoneum covers its anterior surface and sides, while its posterior surface is connected by loose areolar tissue with the left kidney and the origin of the transversus abdominis.
Vascular: The inferior mesenteric artery supplies the descending colon, the sigmoid colon and the superior $\frac{2}{3}$ of the rectum. Venous drainage by the inferior mesenteric vein into the portal system.

I: AXR, CXR (erect): Investigations in an acute presentation.
CT scan: Necessary for planning resections and assessing cancer stage.
Barium enema: May reveal 'apple-core' lesion if tumour present.
Sigmoidoscopy/colonoscopy: For diagnosis of colonic tumours.
Pre-op: Bloods: FBC, U&Es, clotting and crossmatch. Nil by mouth, bowel preparation (if elective), general anaesthetic assessment. Dose of prophylactic antibiotics.
Post-op: NG tube is sometimes used. Maintenance IV fluids with urinary catheter to monitor urine output. An accurate record of fluid balance should be maintained. DVT prophylaxis.

P: Access: Lower midline incision, possibly being extended to full midline incision. Intra-abdominal contents are assessed, e.g. for evidence of enlarged lymph nodes or liver metastases, and the small bowel is packed away from left hemicolon.
Mobilise: The descending colon is mobilised by division of the peritoneal attachments to the level of the splenic flexure. Great care must be taken to avoid injury to the spleen. The transverse colon is mobilised sufficiently to provide a tension-free anastomosis.
Ligation of vessels: Dissection of the sigmoid mesentery is carried out to identify the inferior mesenteric artery branches, which supply the bowel to be resected. These are then isolated, ligated and divided. It is vital to ensure that the arterial supply to the proximal and distal margins are not compromised.
Resection of bowel segment: The bowel is clamped and divided, usually with specialised stapling devices, with removal of segment with the associated mesentery (see Fig. 7b).
Restoration of bowel continuity: An end-to-end anastomosis of the descending colon to the rectosigmoid colon is made if there has been bowel preparation or on-table lavage. This can be accomplished with a special stapling device. Lymph nodes should be sampled in the cases of colonic tumours. A proximal defunctioning stoma may be fashioned to protect the distal anastomosis.
Closure: A pelvic drain is usually left in situ. The abdominal wall is closed with non-absorbable sutures. Skin closure is completed with sutures or clips.

C: Leakage of anastomosis, persistent ileus, ischaemic bowel, peritonitis.

Colorectal resection, Right hemicolectomy

I: **Elective:** Colonic tumours (of the caecum, ascending colon or hepatic flexure) are the most common indications. Rarely, for large carcinoid tumors of the appendix.
Emergency: Occasionally indicated for obstruction, perforation or ischaemia.

A: The ascending colon passes upward from the caecum to the under surface of the right lobe of the liver, where it is lodged in the colic impression. It then bends abruptly forward and to the left, forming the hepatic flexure. The peritoneum covers its anterior surface and sides.
Vascular: Arterial supply derives from branches of the superior mesenteric artery, which consists of the right colic, middle colic and ileocolic artery.

I: **AXR, CXR (erect):** Minimal initial investigations, especially in an emergency.
CT scan: Necessary for planning resections and assessing cancer stage.
Barium enema or colonoscopy: For diagnosis of tumour.
Pre-op: Bloods: FBC, U&Es, clotting, crossmatch. Nil by mouth, bowel preparation, urinary catheterisation, general anaesthetic assessment.
Post-op: NG tube is sometimes used. Urinary catheter and IV fluids with monitoring of fluid balance. DVT prophylaxis.

P: **Access:** Midline (rarely transverse) incision, possibly being extended to full midline incision. Intra-abdominal contents are assessed and the small bowel is packed away.
Mobilise: Lateral peritoneal attachments of the right colon are incised and the colon mobilised. Blunt dissection of the greater omentum is carried out and the transverse colon is divided to mobilise the ascending colon. Careful identification and avoidance of the duodenum, ureter, gonadal vessels.
Ligation of vessels: The mesocolon from the terminal ileum to midtransverse colon is dissected carefully to isolate the ileocolic and right colic vessels that are ligated and divided. The middle colic artery may also be divided if necessary.
Resection of bowel segment: Adequate clearance from the lesion is measured and clamps are placed at the two ends of the length to be resected. The transverse colon and terminal ileum are resected and the resected segment removed (see Fig. 7b).
Restoration of bowel continuity: The terminal ileum is anastomosed to the transverse colon in one or two layers using sutures or staples by end-to-end (most common), end-to-side or side-to-side means. Rarely, an ileostomy may be necessary. Lymph node sampling should be performed in the case of tumours.
Closure: A drain is usually left in situ. The abdominal wall is closed with non-absorbable sutures. Skin closure is completed with sutures or clips.

C: Leakage of anastomosis, persistent ileus, ischaemic bowel, peritonitis.

Colorectal resection, Sigmoid colectomy

Emergency (usually in the form of a Hartmann's procedure): Obstruction, perforation, ischaemic bowel, toxic megacolon.
Elective: Tumours, IBD, diverticular disease.

The sigmoid colon is characterised by an S-shaped loop of variable length joining the descending colon to the rectum at the level of the 3rd sacral segment. It has a mesentery whose root has an inverted V-shaped attachment along the external iliac vessels to the iliac bifurcation and to the anterior sacrum. The left ureter and bifurcation of the common iliac artery lie at the apex of the root.
Vascular: Arterial supply derives from the left colic and sigmoid arteries, and branches of the inferior mesenteric artery. The inferior mesenteric vein returns blood to the portal system.

AXR, CXR (erect): Minimal initial investigations, especially in an emergency.
CT scan: Often necessary for planning resections.
Barium enema: May reveal 'apple-core' lesion or diverticulae.
Sigmoidoscopy: For diagnosis and biopsy.
Pre-op: Nil by mouth, bowel preparation. Bloods: FBC, U&Es, clotting and crossmatch. General anaesthetic assessment.
Post-op: NG tube, IV fluids, DVT prophylaxis. Close monitor of FBC, electrolytes and urine output. Patients' education and support in the management of the stoma if one has been formed.

Access: Lower midline incision, and intra-abdominal contents are assessed. The small bowel is packed away from the sigmoid colon.
Mobilising and ligating vessels: Initial assessement and blunt dissection of the sigmoid mesentery is carried out to identify and ligate supplying vessels. The mesentery is divided with careful identification and avoidance of the ureter and gonadal vessels.
Resection of bowel segment: The sigmoid colon is clamped proximally and distally and the segment resected, usually with stapling devices (see Fig. 7b).
Restoration of bowel continuity:
Hartmann's Procedure: The proximal colon is brought to the surface and an end colostomy is made. The distal bowel is oversewn as a rectal stump. Alternatively, if the distal bowel is long enough, it can be brought out to the abdominal surface to form a mucous fistula.
Anastomosis: This should not be done if there is any risk to the anastomosis from ischaemia or sepsis. Anastomosis can be achieved end-to-end with a single interrupted suture or side-to-side with a stapling device.
Lymph nodes should be sampled in the case of tumours. Peritoneal toilet with extensive washing should be performed if there has been any peritoneal contamination.
Closure: A pelvic drain is usually left in situ. The abdominal wall is closed with non-absorbable sutures. Skin closure is completed with sutures or clips. Following closure of the main wound, the end colostomy is completed in a Hartmann's procecure.

Leakage or breakdown of anastomosis, persistent ileus, ischaemic bowel, peritonitis, breakdown of rectal stump.

D: Injury to the spinal cord with neurological symptoms that depend on the site and extent of injury.

A: Trauma and tumours are the most common causes. Trauma can cause direct cord contusion or compression by bone fragments, haematoma or acute disk prolapses. Tumours can be primary, but are more commonly metastases. Other less common causes are vascular malformations, e.g. cavernous haemangiomas, spinal abscesses and TB (Pott's disease).

A/R: Significant spinal cord injury is assocated with severe trauma, often with head injuries. In the presence of a tumour or vascular malformation, relatively minor trauma can cause severe symptoms. Other predisposing factors include osteoporosis, metabolic bone disease or vertebral disk disease.

E: Common, trauma occurs in all age groups with malignancy or disc disease more common in older ages.

H: History of injury or trauma. Pain, weakness, sensory loss.
Disturbance of bowel or bladder function.
A large central lumbar disk prolapse may cause bilateral sciatica, saddle anaesthesia and urinary retention.
There may be a history of malignancy.

E: Diaphragmatic breathing, reduced anal tone, hyporeflexia, priapism and spinal shock ($\downarrow$ BP without tachycardia) are early signs of a spinal cord injury in trauma.
Sensory: At the level of the lesion.
Motor: Weakness or paralysis (LMN signs) and downward plantar reflexes in the acute phase and at the level of spinal cord injury. UMN signs and upward plantar reflexes in the later phase below the level of spinal cord injury.
Brown-Séquard syndrome: Seen in hemisection of the spinal cord. Below the level of the lesion there is ipsilateral spastic paralysis and loss of postural sense and contralateral loss of pain and thermal sense.

P: The spinal cord exits the skull at the foramen magnum and ends at L1 level, giving rise to 8 cervical, 12 thoracic, 5 lumbar, 5 sacral and 1 coccygeal pairs of spinal nerves. The lumbar, sacral and coccygeal roots form the cauda equina. Useful to remember during examination: C5: shoulder abduction (deltoid); C6: forearm flexion (biceps); C7: forearm extension (triceps); C8: wrist/finger flexion; T1: finger abduction; L2: hip flexion (iliopsoas); L3: knee extension (quadriceps); L4: ankle dorsiflexion (tibialis anterior); S1: ankle plantar flexion (gastrocnemius).

I: **Radiology:** AP and lateral radiographs of cervical (also peg view), thoracic or lumbar spine to look for loss of alignment, loss of height or wedging due to a compression fracture, detached fragments. Emergency MRI or CT scan is necessary in patients suspected of cord injury or compression.
Bloods: FBC, U&Es, Ca^{2+}, ESR, immunoglobulin electrophoresis.
Urine: Bence Jones protein (indicative of multiple myeloma).

M: **Emergency:** Traumatic injuries should be managed according to ATLS guidelines. Following imaging, if a tumour is present, high-dose steroids (dexamethasone) should be given promptly to reduce the oedema and cord compression, or treated with localised radiotherapy. Patients are often transferred to a neurosurgical centre.
Surgery: Surgical stabilisation by external measures, e.g. in the cervical spine, by traction or a halo device or internal stabilisation by bone grafts, or metal implants. Surgical decompression, e.g laminectomy for posterior tumours. Discectomy or microdiscectomy for disc prolapse if symptoms do not settle, or there is an associated neurological deficit.

CONDITIONS

Rehabilitiation: Vital part of management, with multidisciplinary input. May be prolonged in severe injuries.

C: With severe injury or cord transaction there is irreversible loss of spinal function below the level of the lesion. At spinal cord level above C4: respiratory paralysis; C4-T1 quadriplegia, midthoracic: paraplegia; S1: loss of sacral parasympathetic control over bladder and rectum. Of immobility: chest sepsis, urinary sepsis, pressure sores, DVT.

P: Variable depending on the cause and extent of injury. Totally severed nerves or tracts (especially from trauma) rarely recover fully.

I: Triple coronary vessel disease.
Left main stem coronary disease.
Double coronary vessel disease with a proximal left anterior descending artery lesion.

A: The right coronary artery comes off the ascending aorta, runs anteriorly between the pulmonary trunk and right auricle, and then descends along the atrioventricular groove. At the inferior heart border, it passes posteriorly, anastomosing with the left coronary artery. The left coronary artery arises from the ascending aorta, passes posteriorly between the pulmonary trunk and the left auricle into the atrioventricular groove, dividing into the left anterior descending and the left circumflex arteries, which anastomose with the right coronary artery. The internal mammary artery, a branch of the subclavian artery, descends along the pleura behind the costal cartilages ending at the 6th intercostal space where it divides to become the superior epigastric and musculophrenic arteries.

I: **Pre-op:** Patients may have a coronary angiogram, which may indicate the need for surgery. ECG, echocardiogram.
Bloods: FBC, U&Es, clotting and crossmatch. General anaesthetic assessment.
Post-op: Close monitoring in an ITU setting.

P: **Incision:** A midline incision is made down the sternum and the chest wall opened by a median sternotomy. By incising and dissecting open the pericardium, the heart, coronary vessels and great vessels are exposed and inspected.
Obtaining vein graft: The left internal mammary artery is dissected free from the anterior chest wall proximally up to the level of the subclavian vein and distally to its bifurcation. If a leg vein graft is required, an incision is made from the groin to the midcalf to carefully excise and dissect free the long saphenous vein with ligation and division of any branches.
Cardiac bypass: IV systemic heparin is administered. The arterial cannula of the bypass machine is inserted in the ascending aorta for arterial inflow while the venous cannula is inserted and drains the right atrium. The bypass machine cools the blood to 32°C and the aorta is crossclamped proximal to the aortic cannula. A cold cardioplegic solution is administered with topical cooling to induce a hypothermic, cardioplegic arrest. The heart is then maintained at 15–20°C.
Coronary grafting: The distal end of the internal mammary artery is anastomosed distal to an occlusion on either the proximal three-fourths of the left anterior descending artery or proximal circumflex artery due to its limited length. The distal venous bypass graft anastomoses are made by creating a coronary arteriotomy distal to the occlusion and suturing the vein to the opening. The proximal ends of the venous grafts are then anastomosed to the aorta.
Restoration of circulation: The distal vein graft ends are clamped and the aortic clamp removed. Air is extracted from the graft with a needle and syringe to prevent air embolus and the vein clamps are removed. With systemic rewarming, sinus rhythm returns spontaneously or is reinstituted by cardioversion. The patient is gradually taken off the bypass circuit, allowing the heart to fill and resume cardiac ejection.
Closure: On satisfactory cardiac output, all cannulas are removed and protamine is administered. Temporary pacing wires are inserted into the atrium and/or ventricles with two large thoracostomy drains inserted into the pericardium and chest cavity. The sternum is closed with interrupted steel wires and the skin is closed with continuous subcuticular sutures or interrupted sutures.

C: Stroke (2%), intraoperative MI, temporary conduction abnormalities and arrhythmias (e.g. atrial fibrillation), haemorrhage, mediastinitis, wound infection.

P: Operative mortality rate of 3–5%. Left internal mammary artery grafts have a 10-year patency of 90%, whereas venous grafts have a 10-year patency of 50–60%.

CONDITIONS

D: Atherosclerosis of the coronary arteries causing ishcaemic heart disease.

A: Atheroma formation. See **A/R**.

A/R: Hypercholesterolaemia, hypertension, DM, smoking, family history and male gender are all strong risk factors.

E: Common. The leading cause of death in the UK, higher incidence in men than women and prevalence ↑ with age.

H: Asymptomatic in many cases.
History of angina pectoris.
History of MI.

E: May be absent or indicated by signs of risk factors, e.g. arcus in hypercholesterolaemia or signs of consequences, e.g. signs of heart failure.

P: Atherosclerosis of the coronary vessels results in subintimal thickening, formation of atheromatous plaques and luminal narrowing. This leads to restriction in coronary artery blood flow (symptoms of angina) with plaque rupture precipitating thrombus formation and acute vessel occlusion with risk of infarction (acute coronary syndrome).

I: **Stress/Exercise ECG:** Identifies myocardial ischaemia and indicates severity of stenosis; 75% of patients with significant disease will have a positive result.
Stress/Exercise echocardiogram: Shows abnormal myocardial contraction resulting from ischaemia. More sensitive than exercise ECG.
Coronary angiography: Provides accurate anatomical diagnosis and may be combined with angioplasty treatment.

M: **Medical:** See *Rapid Medicine*. Treat symptoms of angina (e.g. nitrates), modify risk factors (e.g. lipid-lowering agent, antihypertensive, diabetic control), reduce risk of MI (aspirin, clopidogrel, heparin, β-blocker).
Coronary angioplasty: Widens or recanalises occluded vessels with intracoronary stents or balloons. Provides good symptom relief but there is still debate about any prognostic advantage over medical therapy. Recent trials suggest that drug-eluting stents (e.g. sirolimus, paclitaxel) reduce restenosis rates.
Surgical: CABG is indicated for symptomatic angina not relieved by medical therapy and in patients with severe three-vessel coronary artery disease, left main stem coronary artery disease or coronary artery disease with impaired left ventricular function.

C: **From disease:** Angina, acute coronary syndromes (ST and non-ST elevation MI), heart failure, valvular disease, cardiac aneurysms, coronary artery disease can raise ASA grade.
From angioplasty: Mortality (3–4%), MI (2%), need for urgent CABG (3–4%), restenosis (30% in 6 months).
From CABG: Mortality (1%), stroke (2%). MI (5–10%).

P: Following CABG, 85–90% of patients gain relief from symptoms of angina, with arterial grafts providing 90% patency at 10 years, whereas vein grafts only 30–50% patency at 10 years.

D: Chronic granulomatous inflammatory disease that can affect any part of the GI tract. Grouped with ulcerative colitis, they are known as IBD.

A: Cause has not yet been elucidated, thought to involve an interplay between genetic and environmental factors.

A/R: **Genetic:** NOD2 gene, HLA-B27 in those with ankylosing spondylitis.
Environmental: Smoking (4–6× risk), refined sugar intake. Link to infectious agents (e.g. mycobacterium) proposed.
Associated with autoimmune diseases (e.g. SLE, autoimmune thyroid disease).

E: Annual UK incidence is 5–8/100 000. Prevalence is 50–80/100 000. Affects any age but peak incidence is in young adults.

H: Crampy abdominal pain (due to transmural and peritoneal inflammation, fibrosis or obstruction of bowel), diarrhoea (may be bloody or steatorrhoea). Fever, malaise, weight loss.
Symptoms of complications.

E: Weight loss, clubbing, signs of anaemia.
Aphthous ulceration of the mouth, perianal skin tags, fistulae and abscesses.
Signs of complications.

P: **Macro:** Inflammation can occur anywhere along GI tract (40% involving the terminal ileum), 'skip' lesions with inflamed segments of bowel interspersed with normal segments. Mucosal oedema and ulceration with 'rose-thorn' fissures (cobblestone mucosa), fistulae, abscesses.
Micro: Transmural chronic inflammation with infiltration of macrophages, lymphocytes and plasma cells. Granulomata with epithelioid giant cells may be seen in blood vessels or lymphatics.

I: **Bloods:** FBC (↓ Hb, ↑ PLTs, ↑ WCC), U&Es, LFT (↓ albumin), ↑ ESR, CRP (↑ or may be normal), haematinics (to look for deficiency states).
Stool microscopy and culture:
AXR: For evidence toxic megacolon.
Erect CXR: If risk of perforation.
Small bowel follow through: May reveal fibrosis or strictures (string sign of Kantor), deep ulceration (rose-thorn), cobblestone mucosa (see Fig. 8).
Endoscopy (OGD, colonoscopy) and biopsy: May help to differentiate between ulcerative colitis and Crohn's disease, useful monitoring for malignancy and disease progression.
Radionuclide-labelled neutrophil scan: Localisation of inflammation (when other tests are contraindicated).

M: **Acute exacerbation:** Fluid resuscitation, IV or oral corticosteroids, antibiotics, analgesia, high-dose 5-ASA analogues, e.g. mesalazine, sulphasalazine may induce a remission in Crohn's disease. DVT prophylaxis is important if unwell. Elemental diet may induce remission (more often used in children). Parenteral nutrition may be necessary.
Monitor: Temperature, pulse, respiratory rate, BP and markers of activity (ESR, CRP, platelets, stool frequency, Hb and albumin). Assess for complications.
Long-term: Steroids for acute exacerbations, regular 5-ASA analogues to ↓ number of relapses in Crohn's colitis. Alternatively, steroid-sparing agents (e.g. azathioprine, 6-mercaptopurine, methotrexate, infliximab).
Advice: Stop smoking, dietitian referral. Education and advice (e.g. from IBD nurse specialists).
Surgery: Indicated for failure of medical treatment, failure to thrive in children, or the presence of complications. This does not prevent recurrence as disease can occur at another GI site.

CONDITIONS

CONDITIONS

C: Gastrointestinal: Haemorrhage, bowel strictures, perforation, fistulae (between bowel, bladder, vagina), perianal fistulae and abscess, GI carcinoma (5% risk in 10 years), malabsorption.
Extraintestinal: Uveitis, episcleritis, gallstones, kidney stones, arthropathy, sacroiliitis, ankylosing spondylitis, erythema nodosum and pyoderma gangrenosum, amyloidosis.

P: Chronic relapsing condition. $\frac{2}{3}$ will require surgery at some stage and $\frac{2}{3}$ of these > 1 surgical procedure. Mortality rate twice that of general population.

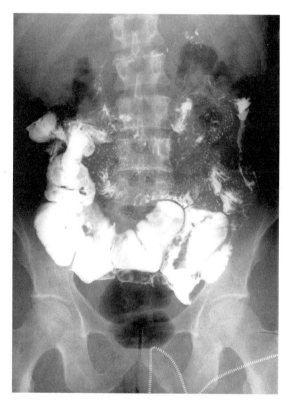

Fig. 8 Crohn's disease.

D: Formation of a thrombus within the deep veins (most commonly of the calf or thigh).

A: Deep veins of the leg are more prone to blood stasis as venous return is dependent on use of surrounding muscles and works against gravity. See **P**athology.

A/R: OCP, post-surgery, prolonged immobility, obesity, pregnancy, dehydration, smoking, polycythaemia, thrombophilia disorders (e.g. deficiency of protein C or antithrombin III), active malignancy.

E: Extremely common. In hospitalised patients, up to 50% have some form of venous stasis.

H: Swollen lower limb. May be painless.

E: **Examining the leg:** Look for local erythema, warmth and swelling. Measure the leg circumference. Look for varicosities and skin coloration changes. Homans' sign should not be performed (passive dorsiflexion of the ankle joint).
Risk stratification: Wells Clinical Prediction Guide:
 – Active cancer
 – Entire leg swelling
 – Recently bedridden for > 3 days or major surgery < 4 weeks
 – Localised tenderness along the distribution of the deep venous system
 – Calf swelling > 3 cm compared to the asymptomatic leg
 – Collateral superficial veins (nonvaricose)
 – Paralysis or recent plaster immobilisation
 – Pitting oedema (greater in the symptomatic leg)
Each of the above scores 1 point. An equally likely alternative diagnosis deducts 2. > 2 is high risk, 1–2 is moderate risk and 0 is low risk.
Examine for PE: Observe respiratory rate, pulse oximetry and pulse rate (see Pulmonary embolism).

P: The mechanisms that lead to vein thrombosis are summed up with **Virchow's triad:**
 (1) Blood vessel wall injury
 (2) Blood flow disturbance (stasis)
 (3) Blood hypercoagulability

I: **Doppler ultrasound:** Gold standard. Good sensitivity for femoral veins, less sensitive for calf veins.
Impedance plethysmography: Changes in blood volume results in changes of electrical resistance of the lower limb. Poor sensitivity for calf veins.
Bloods: None are diagnostic with D-dimers (fibrinogen degradation products) very sensitive but very non-specific and only useful as a negative predictor. If indicated, a thrombophilia screen should be sent. Prior to starting anticoagulation FBC (platelet count prior to starting heparin), U&Es (to check renal function) and clotting.
ECG, CXR and ABG: If there is suggestion that there might be PE, these should be performed. Look for ST, $S_IQ_{III}T_{III}$, axis deviation, hypoxia (see Pulmonary embolism).

M: **Anticoagulation:** Patients should be treated with heparin while awaiting therapeutic INR from warfarin anticoagulation (INR = ~2.5). DVTs not extending above the knee, in some cases may be observed or treated with anticoagulation for 3 months, while those extending beyond the knee require anticoagulation for 6 months. Recurrent DVTs may require long-term warfarin. If active anticoagulation is contraindicated and there is high risk of embolisation, placement of an IVC filter, e.g. Greenfield filter, by interventional radiology is indicated to prevent embolus to the lungs.

CONDITIONS

Prevention: Use of graduated compression stockings. Mobilisation if possible. At-risk groups (immobilised hospital patients) should consider prophylactic heparin, e.g. low molecular weight heparin SC daily (heparin reduces risk to < 10%) if no contraindications.

C: PE. Acutely, it can progress to venous infarction (phlegmasia cerulea dolens). Recurrent DVTs can eventually lead to thrombophlebitis of the deep veins, damage to the valves of the veins and chronic venous insufficiency of the lower limb.

P: Depends on extent of DVT, below-knee DVTs generally have an excellent prognosis, more proximal DVTs are more serious with risk of pulmonary embolus, which if large, may be fatal.

D: Displacement of the femoral head and the complete loss of articulation with the acetabulum. Dislocation can be posterior (90%) or anterior (10%).

A: Trauma.

A/R: There is usually an associated fracture of the acetabulum, femoral shaft, neck or head and sciatic nerve injury following posterior dislocations. Pre-existing disease of the femoral head, acetabulum or neuromuscular system are risk factors for hip dislocation.

E: Occurs commonly in the independent years of life with 70% of all hip dislocations being due to motor vehicle accidents.

H: History of severe trauma. The patient typically complains of severe pain in the hip and upper leg though there may also be knee, lower leg or back pain; is unable to weight bear or move the hip joint; and may have numbness or tingling of the legs in neurovascular injury.

E: **Posterior dislocation:** Shortening, adduction and internal rotation of the affected limb. There may be a drop foot and sensory loss following sciatic nerve injury.
Anterior dislocation: The limb is flexed, abducted and externally rotated with the femoral head being palpable anteriorly.

P: **Posterior dislocation:** The femoral head is dislocated posterior to the acetabulum when the thigh is flexed. The femoral head is either displaced through a tear in the posterior hip capsule or the glenoid lip is avulsed from the acetabulum.
Anterior dislocation: The femoral head is dislocated anteriorly and usually remains lateral to the obturator externus muscle or lies under the iliopsoas muscle in contact with the superior pubic ramus.

I: **Radiographs** (AP, lateral and oblique): To evaluate the location of the femoral head relative to the acetabulum and to exclude any fractures.

M: **Medical:** Strong analgesia.
Surgery: If there are no fractures or there is only a small fracture, closed reduction is performed under general anaesthesia by stabilisation of the pelvis, traction in the line of deformity, flexion of the hip to 90°, then internal followed by external rotation. In irreducible or open dislocations, fractures of the acetabulum and redislocations after reduction, open reduction is performed.
Rehabilitation: The leg is held in traction for 1–2 weeks until the joint is pain-free. Simple movement and exercises are started within 1 week to maintain joint flexibility and the patient is started on crutches after 3 weeks.

C: Fractured acetabulum or femoral head, infection, avascular necrosis of the femoral head, post-traumatic secondary osteoarthritis, recurrent dislocation, sciatic nerve injury.

P: Good to excellent results in about 85% of patients.

CONDITIONS

Dislocation, Shoulder

CONDITIONS

D: Separation of the humeral head from articulation with the scapula. Commonest is anterior dislocation.

A: Falling onto an outstretched hand is the commonest route for anterior dislocations. Posterior dislocations require an adducted arm and can be seen following seizures or electric shock.

A/R: Actions that involve abduction and rotation of shoulder joint have a higher risk of dislocation.

E: Common. Annual incidence is about 17/100 000.

H: History of fall, often onto outstretched hand.
Severe shoulder pain and restricted movement.
There may be a history of previous dislocation.

E: **Anterior shoulder dislocation:**
Arm is held in slight abduction and externally rotated.
Loss of deltoid contour to shoulder.
Humeral head is palpable anteriorly (in the subcoracoid region, beneath the clavicle). Patient resists abduction and internal rotation.
Very important to detect damage to the axillary nerve (with resulting deltoid paralysis) prior to attempt at reduction. Test for sensation in the lateral upper arm 'regimental badge' area.
Posterior shoulder dislocation (uncommon):
Arm is held in adduction and internal rotation.
Anterior shoulder loses contour with prominent coracoid process.
Humeral head palpable beneath the acromion process posteriorly.
Patient resists external rotation and abduction.
Inferior shoulder dislocation (rare):
Arm is fully abducted with elbow commonly flexed on or behind head.
Humeral head may be palpable on the lateral chest wall.

P: Force causes a tear in the joint capsule and displacement of the humeral head, most commonly lying in the infraclavicular fossa, just below the coracoid process.

I: **X-rays of shoulder (AP and scapula view):** Anterior dislocations can be seen as loss of articulation between shoulder and glenoid surface. Posterior dislocations produce a classical 'light bulb' appearance of humeral head on AP view.

M: **Reduction:** Analgesia should be given to reduce pain and muscle spasm. There are many methods but the most commonly used is the external rotation method. While the patient lies supine, adduct the shoulder and flex elbow to 90°. Slowly rotate shoulder externally. Humeral head should 'clunk' into glenoid surface before reaching the coronal plane. Hippocratic and Kocher methods are discouraged as they require application of significant force.
Immobilisation: A shoulder sling is used for immobilisation. The shoulder is reviewed in 1 week.
Recurrent dislocation: Surgery is used to repair the deficient anterior tissues. Putti–Platt operation involves shortening or reefing the subscapularis and Bankart operation involves repair of the capsule and glenoid labrum.

C: Damage to neurovascular structures, most commonly axillary nerve, brachial plexus (posterior cord), radial nerve, brachial artery. Rotator cuff injury. Associated fracture of the humerus.

P: Good. A significant minority of people have 'unstable' shoulder joints that are prone to recurrent dislocations.

D: The clinical condition resulting from the presence of diverticula (outpouchings; see Figs 9a, 9b & 9c) of the colonic mucosa and submucosa through the muscular wall of the large bowel. Diverticulitis is the inflammation of these diverticulae due to impaction of faecalith and pooling of gut flora.

A: A low-fibre, refined diet, common in the West, leads to loss of stool bulk. Consequently, high colonic intraluminal pressures must be generated to propel the stool, leading to herniation of the mucosa and submucosa through the muscularis.

A/R: Low-fibre, refined diet, increasing age, connective tissue disorders.

E: Common, diverticular disease is present in 30–50% of the population > 50 years.

H: Often asymptomatic (80–90%).
Alternating constipation (pellet faeces) and diarrhoea.
GI bleed: PR bleeding may be acute or chronic.
Diverticulitis: Pyrexia and LIF or suprapubic abdominal pain.
Features of complications: For example, pneumaturia, faecaluria and recurrent UTI may be due to a vesico-colic fistula.

E: Usually normal. Occasionally lower abdominal tenderness and faecal loading. If inflammation or abscess development, the patient is unwell, with a tender abdomen; signs of local or generalised peritonitis if perforation has occurred.

P: **Macro:** Diverticulae are most common in the sigmoid and descending colon. Absent from the rectum.
Micro: Diverticulae consist of herniated mucosa and submucosa through the muscularis, particularly at sites of nutrient artery penetration (see Fig. 9c) with a peritoneal covering. There is an associated colonic smooth muscle hypertrophy resulting in luminal stenosis.

I: **Barium enema:** Demonstrates the presence of diverticulae with a saw-tooth appearance of lumen, reflecting smooth muscle hypertrophy (should not be performed if there is a danger of perforation).
Flexible sigmoidoscopy and colonoscopy: Diverticulae can be seen and other pathology (e.g. polyps or tumour) can be excluded.
Bloods: FBC (anaemia), ↑ WCC and ↑ inflammatory markers in acute disease.

M: **GI bleed:** PR bleeding is often managed conservatively with nil by mouth, IV rehydration, antibiotics, blood transfusion if necessary.
Diverticulitis: Nil by mouth, IV antibiotics (cephalosporin and metronidazole) and IV fluid rehydration.
Chronic: High-fibre diet with bulking agent (e.g. methylcellulose). Laxatives may be required if constipation is severe. Encourage high fluid intake.
Surgery: May be necessary with recurrent attacks or when complications develop, e.g. severe bleeding or infection. Sigmoid colectomy, Hartmann's procedure, fistulectomy or drainage of pericolic abscesses are some operations performed.

C: Diverticulitis, pericolic abscess, perforation, colonic obstruction, fistula formation (bladder, small intestine, vagina), haemorrhage (caused by vessel erosion).

P: 10–25% of patients will have one episode of diverticulitis. Of these, 30% will have a second episode. 20% of patients will have one or more complication after the first episode of diverticulitis.

CONDITIONS

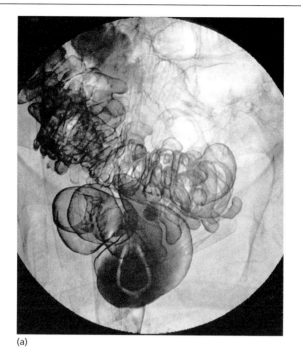

(a)

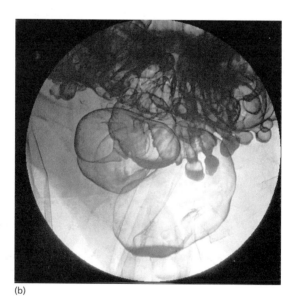

(b)

Fig. 9 (a & b) Both figures show severe diverticular disease.

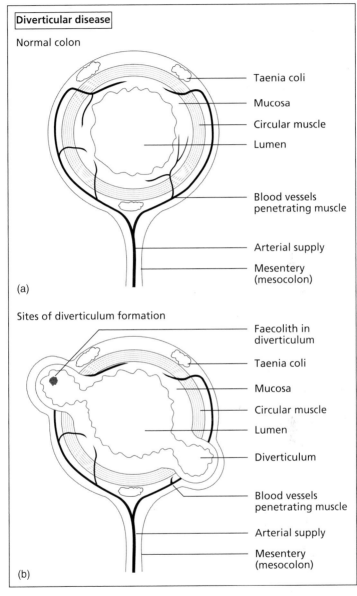

Diverticular disease

Normal colon

- Taenia coli
- Mucosa
- Circular muscle
- Lumen

- Blood vessels penetrating muscle

- Arterial supply

- Mesentery (mesocolon)

(a)

Sites of diverticulum formation

- Faecolith in diverticulum
- Taenia coli
- Mucosa
- Circular muscle
- Lumen
- Diverticulum

- Blood vessels penetrating muscle

- Arterial supply

- Mesentery (mesocolon)

(b)

CONDITIONS

Fig. 9c

CONDITIONS

D: Mononeuropathies caused by nerve compression from surrounding structures.

A: **Carpal tunnel syndrome:** Compression of the median nerve within the carpal tunnel of the hand. Predisposing factors include pregnancy, hypothyroidism, acromegaly and wrist joint disease.
Ulnar nerve entrapment: Compression of the ulnar nerve as it passes along the ulnar groove behind the medial epicondyle of the humerus. Predisposing factors include arthritis of the elbow joint, previous supracondylar fractures.
Meralgia paraesthetica: Lateral cutaneous nerve of the thigh may be compressed by the inguinal ligament in pregnancy, obesity or tight trousers.
Common peroneal compression: Compression of the common peroneal nerve as it winds around the neck of the fibula. Common mechanisms is with plaster casts, proximal fibula fractures.
Facial nerve compression: Mass in parotid gland, mass in the auditory canal.

A/R: See **A**.

E: Common. Carpal tunnel is 8× more common in females.

H: Sensory changes in distribution of nerve, pins and needles, numbness, pain.
Carpal tunnel: Median nerve (radial $3\frac{1}{2}$ digits of the hand), often worse at night and exacerbated by certain tasks, e.g. typing.
Ulnar nerve: Ulnar nerve (last $1\frac{1}{2}$ digits of the hand).
Meralgia paraesthetica: sensory disturbance over anterolateral aspect of thigh.
Common peroneal compression: Dorsum of foot may have impaired sensation.

E: Putting pressure on the site of nerve compression may bring on or worsen the symptoms. Sensory impairment in the affected nerve distribution.
Weakness, wasting (if prolonged) of muscles in affected nerve distribution (e.g. thenar eminence muscles in carpal tunnel syndrome).
Carpal tunnel syndrome: Tapping over the carpal tunnel (Tinel's test), hyperflexing of the wrists for 1 min (Phalen's test) reproduces symptoms.
An important differential is C6-C7 radiculopathy, suggested by other motor signs (e.g. brachioradialis weakness, loss of triceps reflex or sensory involvement of the palm of the hand or forearm).
Ulnar nerve: Weakness of long finger flexors and intrinsic muscles of the hand, the end result would be a 'claw hand'. Sensory impairment in the fifth finger and ulnar border of the hand.
Common peroneal nerve: Foot drop, sensory disturbance of the leg and dorsum of foot. There may be weakness of ankle eversion but there is preserved ankle inversion (sparing of tibialis posterior) and preserved ankle reflex. Main differential is L5 radiculopathy (where ankle inversion is affected).

P: Nerve compression can result in nerve ischaemia and segmental demyelination (neuropraxia), which can eventually cause axonal degeneration.

I: **Nerve conduction studies:** Often unnecessary but allows confirmation.
Bloods: TFT, glucose (diabetes can cause mononeuropathies), ESR.

M: **Carpal tunnel syndrome:** Nonsurgical measures include steroid injections into the carpal tunnel, wrist splints and treatment of cause. Surgical decompression consists of division of the flexor retinaculum.
Ulnar nerve: Conservative management or surgical release of the nerve from the ulnar groove, resiting the course anterior to the medial epicondyle (anterior nerve transposition).
Meralgia paraesthetica: Encourage weight loss, avoid tight clothing.
Common peroneal compression: Conservative approach often results in recovery; however, exploration and decompression may be required.
Facial nerve compression: Excision of cause (e.g. parotid gland mass).

C: Recurrence following conservative measures is common. Irreversible loss of nerve function if progressive compression with weakness, wasting and sensory loss.

P: Depends on cause and treatment, but persistent symptoms are not uncommon.

CONDITIONS

D: Inflammation of the epididymis or testes (orchitis). 60% of epididymitis are associated with orchitis and most cases of orchitis with epididymitis.

A: Majority of cases are infective in origin.
Bacterial: < 35 years most commonly *Chlamydia* or *Gonococcus*. > 35 years most common are coliforms. Rare: TB, syphilis.
Viral: Mumps can cause orchitis.
Fungal: Candida if immunocompromised.
1/3 are idiopathic. May be associated with underlying testicular tumour.

A/R: Diabetes. Rarely associated with vasculitis, e.g. Henoch–Schönlein purpura. Also with urethral instrumentation and prostatic surgery.

E: Common. Affects all age groups, 50% are 20–30 years.

H: Painful, swollen and tender testes or epididymis (usually unilateral), onset is usually less acute than testicular torsion – the most important differential. Penile discharge may occur (especially in bacterial forms), fever. Important to enquire about sexual history.

E: Swollen and tender epididymis and/or testis.
The scrotum may be erythematous and oedematous.
Pyrexia.
Walking or even eliciting a cremaster reflex may be painful.

P: The epididymis is an elongated mass of convoluted efferent tubes posterior and superior to the testes. Spermatozoa mature and gain their mobility within this structure.

I: **Urine:** Dipstick, early morning urine collection (bacterial C&S and microscopy for acid-fast bacilli if TB suspected).
Blood: FBC, ↑ WCC, ↑ CRP, U&Es.
Imaging: ↑ Blood flow on Duplex examination, ultrasound may reveal local collection or abscess.
Following treatment of acute episode, older patients should be investigated for causes of bladder outlet obstruction, e.g. flow studies or underlying malignancy.

M: **Medical:** Antibiotic treatment, if severe may need IV treatment initially. Young patients where chlamydia is likely, doxycycline for 2 weeks and attendance as a genitourinary clinic for follow-up and contact tracing. In older patients, quinolones (e.g. ciprofloxacin) are recommended for 2–4 weeks. Adequate analgesic and scrotal support. Follow-up is still recommended to exclude testicular malignancy. If TB is suspected, antituberculous regimen is necessary.
Surgical: Exploration of scrotum if testicular torsion cannot be excluded or if an abscess develops that requires drainage. Also performed in cases of tuberculous epididymo-orchitis not responding to medical treatment.

C: Pain, abscess; if untreated, risk of spreading infection and Fournier's gangrene. Minimal risk to fertility if unilateral and treated. Mumps orchitis may cause testicular atrophy and future fertility problems.

P: Good if treated. May take up to 2 months for swelling to completely resolve.

Extradural haemorrhage

D: Bleeding and accumulation of blood into the extradural space.

A: Trauma, most commonly fractures of the temporal or parietal bones causing rupture of the middle meningeal artery.

A/R: Risk factors are haemorrhagic diathesis (e.g. haemophilia, anticoagulation therapy), dural vascular anomalies (e.g. dural AVMs).

E: Annual incidence of 20/100 000 in the UK. 10% of severe head injuries. Most commonly seen in young adults. Uncommon in elderly (subdural haemorrhages are more common in that age group).

H: Head injury with a temporary loss of consciousness, followed by a lucid interval, then development of progressive deterioration in conscious level.

E: Signs of scalp trauma or fracture.
Headache.
Deteriorating GCS, signs of raised ICP (e.g. dilated unresponsive pupil on the side of the injury).
Rising BP and bradycardia (Cushing's reflex) is a late sign.

P: Trauma causes a fracture, most commonly of the squamous temporal bone as this is the thinnest part of the cranial vault. This can rupture the middle meningeal artery, with the arterial bleeding causing rapid accumulation of blood and stripping the dura from the inner table of the skull. This results in raised ICP and compression of the underlying brain parenchyma.

I: **Urgent CT scan:** Diagnostic and identifies location of haematoma. An arterial bleed produces a convex or lens-shaped haematoma. Associated signs of raised ICP include midline shift, compression of ventricles, obliteration of basal cisterns sulcal effacement.

M: **Early management of head injuries:** Following ATLS guidelines, which requires establishing ABC and cervical spine control. Once stabilised, assessment is made of severity of head injury with an urgent CT scan.
Surgical: Urgent craniotomy and decompressive evacuation of the haematoma with diathermy or clipping of source of bleeding. An ICP monitor may be placed for post-op monitoring. Close observation and supportive care is required, often in an ITU setting.

C: Acutely, the greatest risk is cerebral herniation and death. In the longer term, neurobehavioural changes (e.g. postconcussive syndrome, retrograde amnesia).

P: Mortality rates relate to initial GCS and associated intracerebral injuries. If treated early, prognosis is good with underlying brain usually suffering limited injury.

D: The abnormal protrustion of a peritoneal sac, often with abdominal contents, through the femoral canal.

A: The predisposing factor is the anatomy of the femoral canal with distinct unyielding boundaries of medially the lacunar ligament, anteriorly the inguinal ligament, posteriorly the pectineal ligament and pubic bone, and laterally the femoral vein. The canal only usually consists of loose connective tissue and lymph node (Cloquet's node).

A/R: Females (have a wider angle between the inguinal ligament and pectineal part of the pubic bone and a wider femoral canal), pregnancy, raised intra-abdominal pressure (heavy lifting, cough or straining due to constipation or prostatism).

E: $25\times$ less common than inguinal hernias, female : male is 4 : 1.

H: As femoral hernias are often small, they often go unnoticed until they become strangulated or obstructed, presenting as a surgical emergency (up to 80%) with symptoms of pain, abdominal distention, nausea, vomiting, absolute constipation. Also presents with lower abdominal discomfort, or lump or bulge in the groin region.

E: Careful inspection will show a swelling in the groin below and lateral to the pubic tubercle (although if large, may tend to spread up and over the inguinal ligament).
There is absence of a cough impulse over the inguinal ring. If incarcerated or strangulated, the hernia may be very tender.
Signs of bowel obstruction (e.g. distension, high pitched bowel sounds).
Other differentials include inguinal hernia, lymphadenopathy, hydrocoele or lipoma of the spermatic cord, groin or psoas abscess, saphaena varix or femoral aneurysm.

P: The narrow margins of the femoral canal predispose to incarceration of the hernia contents that could consist of omentum, bowel, extraperitoneal fat or other organs such as ovary. The vascular supply becomes compromised and involved tissues become ischaemic and gangrenous if the hernia is not operated on promptly.

I: **Bloods:** FBC, U&Es, clotting, G&S, ABG (for metabolic acidosis in bowel ischaemia).
Imaging: AXR: may show SBO, USS if a different diagnosis is suspected, but should not delay surgery if an incarcerated hernia is suspected.

M: **Emergency:** Resuscition is very important, with attention to rehydration and correction of electrolyte imbalances, placement of an NG tube if vomiting, antibiotics if signs of sepsis and surgical repair as definitive treatment.
Surgery: Principles involve dissection of the sac, observing and reducing the contents, excising the sac and repairing the defect, usually by approximation of the inguinal and pectineal ligaments using non-absorbable sutures. Three approaches:
(1) *Low (Lockwood)* transverse incision over the hernia.
(2) *Transinguinal (Lotheissen)* incision above and parallel to the inguinal ligament, through the external oblique, inguinal canal and transversalis fascia (may have a higher recurrence rate).
(3) *High (McEvedy)* approach using an oblique, paramedial or unilateral Pfannenstiel incision, opening the rectus sheath, retracting rectus medially and dividing transversalis to expose the femoral canal. This is used if strangulation is suspected. The sac is opened and contents inspected. If viable, they are reduced or if nonviable bowel is present, this is resected (may necessitate a lower midline incision if a high approach is not used).

CONDITIONS

C: Femoral hernias commonly strangulate, resulting in bowel obstruction, ischaemia and gangrene, which may necessitate surgical resection.
Of surgery: The lacunar ligament can be incised, occasionally causing bleeding from an aberrant obturator artery running medially.

P: Outcome is generally good with prompt and appropriate surgery, recurrence after repair is uncommon ($< 3\%$).

D: Fracture of bones forming the osseoligamentous mortise of the ankle joint.
Unimalleolar fractures involve only one malleolus (usually lateral) (see Fig. 10b).
Bimalleolar (Pott) fractures involve two malleoli (usually medial and lateral).
Trimalleolar (Cotton) fractures involve the medial, lateral, and posterior malleoli (posterior lip of articular surface of tibia) (see Fig. 10a).
Pilon fractures are those of the distal tibia metaphysis that extend into the ankle joint and are commonly associated with a distal fibula fracture.

A: Trauma (e.g. direct, indirect or rotational), pathological.

A/R: Commonly associated with collateral ligament injuries or ankle subluxation or dislocation, or fractures of the proximal fibula, base of 5th metatarsal, calcaneus or navicular.

E: Very common.

H: Enquire in detail about the mechanism of the injury, inversion or eversion injury, whether able to bear weight after the injury, and any history of previous trauma to the ankle.

E: For presence of an open wound, swelling, erythema, bony tenderness. Assess the range of motion, ligamentous laxity and neurovascular status.

P: The distal tibia, distal fibula, talus and calcaneus provide the joint framework.
Danis–Weber classification of ankle fractures uses the position of the level of the fibular fracture relative to the syndesmosis:
Type A: Fracture below the syndesmosis.
Type B: Fracture at the level of the syndesmosis, with the tibiofibular ligaments usually intact.
Type C: Fracture above the syndesmosis, which tears the syndesmosis ligaments.
Lauge–Hansen classification uses two-word descriptors: the first describes the position of the foot, and the second describes the motion of the foot (talus) with respect to the leg. Categories include supination-adduction, supination-eversion, pronation-abduction, pronation-eversion and pronation-dorsiflexion.

I: The Ottawa ankle rules for X-ray include the inability to bear weight immediately after the injury or at the time of presentation, and tenderness over the posterior surface or tip of malleoli.
Radiographs: Should include AP, lateral and mortise views. The fibula should also be imaged if there is proximal fibula tenderness.

M: **Fracture dislocations:** Should be reduced and immobilised prior to X-ray to prevent skin necrosis over the medial malleolus.
Closed reduction and splint: For simple uncomplicated lateral malleolar fractures.
Open reduction, internal fixation: Indicated for pilon, bimalleolar and trimalleolar fractures, or lateral malleoli fractures with damage to the deltoid ligament (>5 mm on X-ray with ankle on eversion).
Open fractures: Should be treated urgently. Protect from further contamination by covering wounds with a wet, sterile dressing secured by loosely wrapped dry sterile gauze. Consider antibiotic prophylaxis, tetanus immunisation. May need temporary external fixation prior to definitive fixation and soft tissue cover.
Rehabilitation: Always avoid immobilisation of the ankle in equines. After swelling subsides and evidence of healing, encourage weightbearing.

C: Non-union or mal-union of the fracture. Chronic persistent symptoms (e.g. pain, weakness and instability of the ankle) may develop. Traumatic arthritis complicates 20–40% of ankle fractures. In children, ankle fractures involving the growth plate may cause chronic deformity with disturbance of growth of the limb.

P: Isolated, nondisplaced lateral malleolus fracture (the most common ankle fracture) has a favourable prognosis.

CONDITIONS

CONDITIONS

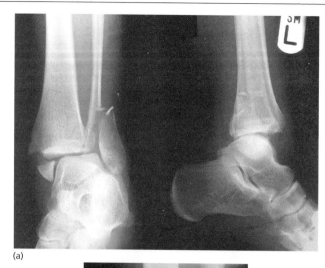
(a)

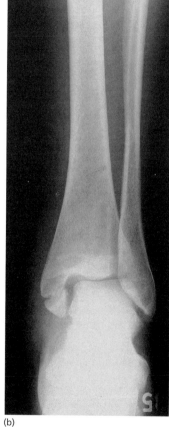
(b)

Fig. 10 (a) Trimalleolar fracture of the left ankle; (b) fracture of the left medial malleolus.

D: A break in the continuity of the cortex of the clavicle.

A: Indirect trauma to the shoulder or clavicle. Classically, due to fall onto an outstretched arm or onto the shoulder.

A/R: Risk factors include osteoporosis and seizures.

E: Extremely common.

H: History of trauma to shoulder.
Painful shoulder on movement.

E: Of peripheral pulses, distal neurology and neighbouring joints.
Tender shoulder joint or around the site of the fracture.
Loss of prominence of the clavicle on inspection.

P: The clavicle is an S-shaped bone that articulates with the sternum medially and the acromion process laterally. Most fractures of the clavicle are at the junction of the middle and outer 1/3. Displacement of the lateral fragment inferiorly and medially is common. As the subclavian vein lies directly under (around 1 cm medial from the midpoint), it is at risk of damage. The brachial plexus also lies beneath it but on the lateral third.

I: **Radiographs:** AP and oblique clavicle views.

M: **Conservative:** Nonsurgical management, with use of simple analgesic and arm support, using either a simple or figure-of-eight sling for ~2 weeks. Shoulder exercises should be carried out as soon as the pain settles to prevent stiffness.
Internal fixation: Rarely indicated except in open fractures or gross dislocation. Usually for distal 1/3 fractures where non-union is more likely to occur. Plate fixation is the commonest method.

C: Injury to the subclavian vein or the brachial plexus (usually the medial cord).
Floating shoulder: If occurring with a scapular fracture, this is known as 'floating shoulder', where deformity is more likely to be greater as the upper limb is no longer articulated with the thorax.
Long-term: Mal-union, shoulder stiffness, non-union.

P: Good, and most clavicular fractures unite and heal rapidly. Non-union in conservative treatment is < 1%. There is usually some callus formation, which can be quite prominent, but there is usually little to no loss of function.

CONDITIONS

CONDITIONS

D: Fractures of the metacarpal or phalangeal bones.

A: Trauma.

A/R: Sporting activities, fights, accidents.

E: Common, incidence $\sim$ 380/100 000 in the UK.

H: Handedness should be noted. History of mechanism of injury, e.g. direct trauma, punching. Area of pain and loss of function should be noted.

E: Look for localised tenderness, swelling, open wounds, especially that may have been created by teeth. Signs of pain and $\downarrow$ range of movement, crepitus or deformity, e.g. dorsal lump in metacarpal shaft fractures, knuckle flattening in metacarpal neck fractures, shortening of the thumb in Bennett's fracture. Examine neurovascular status of involved area.

P: **Metacarpal fractures:** Shaft fractures are common, often of the little/ring fingers with the distal fragment that may flex on the palmar side. Metacarpal little finger neck fracture – 'boxer's fracture' – is the most common hand fracture. Exclude rotational deformity. Metacarpal base fractures (excluding thumb base) are usually stable fractures.
Bennett's fracture: An oblique fracture involving the carpometacarpal joint of the thumb base with proximal subluxation of the distal fragment.
Proximal or middle phalangeal fracture: Usually a transverse or short oblique fracture, angulate into extension. An angulated force can result in intra-articular bone fracture. Can be associated with damage to tendon sheaths.
Terminal phalangeal fracture: Usually from a direct blow, often shattering the bone into fragments.
Mallet finger: A fragment of the terminal phalangeal base is avulsed off by the extensor tendon resulting in the loss of active extension of the distal interphalangeal joint.

I: **X-ray of the digit, hand or wrist:** Focusing on area of clinical suspicion.

M: **Initial:** Splinting and analgesic, e.g. buddy strapping of digits, metacarpal fractures should be splinted in the 'Edinburgh' position. Wound toilet with irrigation and suturing if indicated. Tetanus booster if required. Open fractures should be treated with antibiotics. Early referral to orthopaedic clinic.
Conservative: Advice on hand elevation, mobilisation usually within 3 weeks. A boxer's fracture is treated this way with operative intervention rarely required. Most injuries to the metacarpal are managed with closed reduction and external splint immobilisation.
Surgery: Indications for operative treatment include failure to achieve or maintain acceptable reduction, open fractures, multiple fractures in the hand, complex injuries, displaced intra-articular injuries, and fractures with serious soft tissue injury requiring stable skeletal support. Restoration of function is the prime aim. Internal fixation with Kirschner wires for large displacements, unstable fractures, intra-articular fractures and irreducible fractures. External fixation for open or comminuted fractures with significant soft tissue injury.

C: Metacarpal fractures: metacarpalgia (pain on gripping), dorsal swelling. Malunion, stiffness and rarely non-union.

P: Most fractures will heal in about 3–6 weeks with good recovery of function.

D: A break in the continuity of the cortex of the humerus.

A: Direct or indirect trauma to the humerus (e.g. fall onto elbow or onto out-stretched hand). The trauma may be trivial if there is an underlying pathology. A twisting injury to the arm may cause a spiral shaft fracture, or in children should raise suspicion of non-accidental injury.

A/R: Predisposing factors to a fracture include bony metastases, primary bone tumours, osteoporosis, osteomalacia.

E: Common. 1% of all fractures are humeral fractures.

H: History of trauma to upper limb.
Pain on use of upper limb.
Wrist drop (from extensor muscle weakness supplied by the radial nerve).

E: Painful upper limb, especially on motion of the shoulder joint.
Assess for associated nerve damage, e.g. loss of sensation on the dorsal aspect of the hand (radial nerve damage).
Examine peripheral pulses to assess for vascular damage.
Always examine for other fractures (e.g. clavicle, skull, pelvis, limbs).

P: **Anatomy:** The humeral head articulates with the glenoid cavity of the scap-ula. The head is connected to the shaft by the surgical neck lying between two tubercles. The surgical neck is frequently the site of fracture. The radial sulcus winds down along the shaft of the humerus carrying the radial nerve and the profunda artery.
Neer classification of proximal humeral fractures: Classified by the number of displaced main fragments.

I: **X-rays of humerus (AP and lateral views), elbow and shoulder:** Allows confirmation of location of fractures and any predisposing lesions (see Fig. 11).
Bloods: Unnecessary for uncomplicated fractures.

M: **Conservative:** Suitable for isolated uncomplicated fractures (e.g. closed or undisplaced). Functional bracing with collar and cuff for humeral neck frac-tures, or plaster-of-Paris cast for shaft fractures.
Surgical: Indicated for compound, open, displaced or pathological fractures or associated neurovascular injury. Open reduction and internal fixation for dis-placed two- or three-part proximal humerus fractures. Four-part fractures may require hemiarthroplasty. Humeral shaft fractures may be treated by intrame-dullary nailing, plating or external fixation.

C: Radial nerve damage occurs in about 10% of cases, with loss of wrist and finger extension. Shoulder or elbow stiffness is common. If severe, avascular necrosis of the humeral head.

P: Good recovery for uncomplicated fractures. Radial nerve function returns in 3–4 months if due to a neuropraxia in majority of patients.

CONDITIONS

CONDITIONS

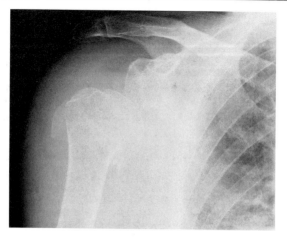

Fig. 11 Fracture of the head of right humerus.

D: Break in the continuity of cortical bone of the femur at or above the lesser trochanter.

A: Often follows a fall with a backround of ↓ bone mass (see below).

A/R: Most commonly due to osteoporosis and ↑ prevalence of falls in elderly, other risk factors are current smoking, ↓ BMI (< 18.5), previous low trauma fracture after 50 years of age and maternal history of hip fracture. Others include hyperparathyroidism, metastases, Paget's disease.

E: Common in the elderly, with lifetime risk of 18% in women, 6% in males (female : male is 4 : 1). Prevalence 3/100 (65–74 years), 12.6/100 (> 85 years).

H: History of fall, may be minor, resulting in pain and restriction of movement in the hip area. Premorbid mobility, mental status and general health should be noted.

E: The affected leg is shortened, adducted and externally rotated, with pain in the hip.

P: Fractures are classified into two categories:
Intracapsular: Occur proximal to the point where the hip joint capsule attaches to the femur; includes subcapital, transcervical and basicervical.
Extracapsular: Trochanteric (see Fig. 12a & 12b) or subtrochanteric.
Can be subdivided into **undisplaced** and **displaced**.
As the principle blood supply to the femoral head is via retinacular vessels that travel back along the capsule, intracapsular fractures can interrupt supply and result in avascular necrosis.

I: **Bloods:** FBC, U&Es, clotting, G&S.
Imaging: Plain radiographs AP and lateral views of the hip. If there is doubt regarding diagnosis, MRI, bone scan or repeat plain radiographs after a delay of 24–48 h should be performed. CXR if elderly and surgery required.

M: **Prevention:** Risk assessment and interventions aimed at reducing risk of falls. Hip protectors have been shown to be beneficial.
Medical: Calcium, vitamin D, HRT, selective oestrogen receptor modulators, bisphosphonates, calcitonin, fluoride and thiazides have been used for primary or secondary prevention.
Immediate: Resuscitation, correction of fluid and electrolyte imbalance, analgesia and attention to pressure areas. Patients should be operated on within 24 h, as this reduces the risk of thrombotic complications and pressure damage.
Undisplaced intracapsular fractures: Internal fixation allows early mobilisation and reduces risk of fractures becoming displaced; in the very elderly, hemiarthroplasty may be considered.
Displaced intracapsular fractures: Open reduction and internal fixation (younger, more active patients), hemiarthroplasty or total hip replacement (may be appropriate in patients with pre-existing joint disease, good activity levels and a reasonable life expectancy).
Extracapsular fractures: Should be treated surgically unless medical contra-indication by reduction and internal fixation using extramedullary (e.g. sliding screw and plate) or intramedullary (e.g. Gamma nail implants).
All patients should receive antibiotic prophylaxis at induction and DVT prophylaxis.

C: **Early:** Pain, immobility, infections, DVT (asymptomatic up to 45%, symptomatic up to 11%) and PE (3–13%), pressure sores (20%), pulmonary complications (ARDS, fat embolism, pneumonia).
Late: Avascular necrosis of the femoral head, non-union, and implant failure.

P: Mortality after hip fracture is high, 30% at 1 year, with 25% requiring a higher level of long-term care.

CONDITIONS

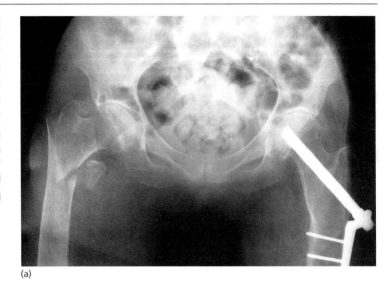

(a)

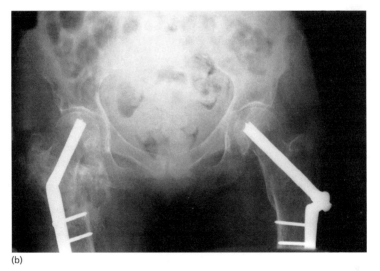

(b)

Fig. 12   (a) A right trochanteric (extracapsular) fracture. (b) Same patient post-reduction and internal fixation with a dynamic hip screw.

D: A break in the continuity of the cortex of the ribs.

A: Blunt trauma to the chest (e.g. fall, driver impact with steering wheel). Fractures in children may raise suspicion of non-accidental injury.

A/R: Often associated with polytrauma. Predisposing factors include bony metastases, osteoporosis, osteomalacia.

E: Common.

H: Enquire about history and nature of trauma. Chest wall pain, worse on inspiration, coughing, moving. Dyspnoea.

E: Localised chest wall tenderness with bruising. Look for paradoxical chest wall movement suggestive of flail chest (segment of chest wall rises with expiration and depresses with inspiration). Tachypnoea and cyanosis suggest complications. **Pneumothorax or haemothorax:** Reduced air entry on affected side. Hyper- or hyporesonant on affected side. Tracheal deviation away from affected side. Always examine for other fractures (e.g. clavicle, skull, pelvis, limbs).

P: Fractures most often occur near the angle of the rib and, due to associated muscular and ligamentous attachments, are rarely severely displaced. Nevertheless, may cause surrounding damage resulting in pneumo- or haemothorax.

I: **Imaging: CXR:** Allows confirmation of location of fractures and any predisposing lesions. Also, examine for pneumothorax. Lateral films and expiratory films may also be considered. CT chest if severe injury once stabilised. **Bloods:** Unnecessary for uncomplicated fractures. Others as indicated in severe trauma, e.g. FBC. U&Es, clotting, G&S, crossmatch, ABG.

M: **Conservative** (for isolated uncomplicated fractures of <3 ribs)**:** Simple analgesic and advice on breathing exercises to prevent chest infection. **Associated with severe trauma:** Managed according to ATLS guidelines. If there is an associated pneumo- or haemothorax, high-flow oxygen. For tension pneumothorax, urgent needle decompression may be necessary. A chest drain insertion should be considered if >20% or if there is respiratory compromise. For haemothorax, patient should also receive fluid and blood resuscitation. Coagulopathies need to be corrected urgently. Cardiothoracic surgery may be necessary if bleeding persists. **Flail chest:** High-flow oxygen. Best managed in ITU, and may require tracheal intubation for intermittent positive pressure ventilation.

C: **Early:** Pneumothorax, haemothorax, pulmonary contusions, flail chest (if three or more ribs have fractures in more than two places, where a segment of the chest wall becomes capable of independent movement). **Later:** Pneumonia, injury to long thoracic nerve.

P: Good recovery for uncomplicated fractures. Potentially high mortality for complicated fractures if not diagnosed and managed early.

CONDITIONS

CONDITIONS

D: A break in the continuity of the tibia and/or fibula.

A: Trauma (direct, indirect or rotational), pathological (fractures that occur in the absence of significant force).

A/R: Fractures of the tibia generally are associated with fibula fracture, because the force is transmitted along the interosseous membrane to the fibula.

E: Common, in active young population or in the elderly who are prone to falls.

H: History of direct or indirect trauma, pain, swelling, and inability to mobilise with tibia fracture. Mobilisation is possible with isolated fibula fracture.

E: Inspect for obvious deformity. Examine the ankle and knee joint for any associated fractures.
Common peroneal nerve injury is not uncommon, especially with high fractures of the fibula. This presents as foot drop and loss of sensation over the lateral aspect of the dorsal foot. There is preservation of power in foot inversion.

P: The tibia articulates with the femur superiorly (in the knee joint) and the talus inferiorly. Its inferior prominence is the medial malleolus. The posterior tibial artery and nerve run along posteromedially and wind around the medial malleolus to enter the foot.
The fibula connects to the tibia superiorly and medially (via the interosseous membrane), and articulates with the talus inferiorly. Its inferior prominence is the lateral malleolus. The common peroneal nerve runs around the groove at the fibular neck and divides into the deep and superifical peroneal nerves. These supply the peroneal muscles and the extensor compartment of the lower limb.

I: **Bloods:** FBC, G&S (in severe trauma).
Radiographs: AP and lateral views are sufficient to diagnose fractures. Look for displacement of bone. Technetium bone scan is more sensitive for detection of stress fractures.

M: **Medical:** Analgesia, tetanus prophylaxis and broad-spectrum antibiotic coverage for open fractures. Fluids and blood transfusion may be needed if there is significant blood loss.
Surgical: Closed reduction and external immobilisation may be suitable in some fractures. For isolated midshaft or proximal fibula fracture, 5–7 days without weightbearing activity resolves most of the swelling to allow weightbearing activity. Open fractures, which extend to nearby articular surfaces, require open reduction and internal fixation. This usually involves an intramedullary nail or external pins.

C: Limb loss as a result of severe soft tissue trauma, neurological or vascular deficit, compartment syndrome, infection. Injury to the common peroneal nerve. Delayed union, and non-union.

P: Good for uncomplicated fractures. High risk of mal-union if the fracture displacement is > 50%.

D: Break in the continuity of the vertebrae.

A: Trauma, underlying pathogical bone.

A/R: Risk factors include osteoporosis, bony metastases, osteomyelitis.

E: Very common. In the younger individual (mostly male) due to trauma, accidents or falls. A second peak is in the elderly, usually secondary underlying bony pathology.

P: Vertebral fractures can be divided according to the mechanism of injury.
Forced flexion (most common) of the spine results in a wedge fracture of the vertebral body. Normally stable but torn posterior ligaments can cause instability.
Hyperextension of the head causes anterior ligament injury, intervertebral disc damage or neural arch fracture. Usually stable except for C-2 pedicle fractures ('Hangman's fracture').
Axial compression from a vertical force on the spine leads to a vertical vertebral fracture complicated by disc material being forced into the vertebral body, driving bony fragments into the spinal canal (burst fractures).
Flexion, compression and posterior distraction damages the posterior and middle segments of the spine, displacing bone fragments and disc material into the spinal canal. This is an unstable fracture.
Flexion, rotation and shear leads to rupture of ligaments and joint capsule, facet fractures, shearing off of the top of a vertebra and the above vertebra dislocating forwards. Always unstable and high incidence of neurological damage.
Horizontal translation is an unstable fracture with a very high risk of neural damage due to the vertebral column splitting with one segment translating laterally or anteroposteriorly.

H: History of trauma and the mechanism of injury. Complaint of pain or stiffness of the neck or spine. Numbness, paraesthesiae, weakness or loss of sphincter control may occur with neural damage.

E: Localised tenderness, bruising or haematoma. Sensorimotor deficits from neurological damage.

I: **X-rays (AP and lateral views) of the affected spine** to identify the fracture. The 3-column theory states that a fracture is unstable if 2 out of 3 columns are disrupted. These theoretical columns are the anterior vertebral body, the posterior vertebral body and the vertebral arch.
CT scan: Shows vertebral body or neural arch fractures.
MRI scan: Images spinal cord (for compression) and soft tissue lesions.

M: **According to ATLS guidelines in trauma.**
Conservative: For stable fractures. Reduction of any dislocation or subluxation by traction or adjusting posture. Use of a firm collar or a brace for stable fractures. Bed rest and analgesia until pain and muscle spasm subsides.
Surgery: A halo-body cast is used for unstable cervical fractures, whereas internal fixation with bone grafts, plates or wires is used in unstable thoracolumbar fractures. Decompression is necessary for any bone fragments encroaching the spinal canal. Spinal fusion is needed for burst fractures threatening the spinal cord.
Rehabilitation: Required for any neurological deficit.

C: Death, spinal cord damage, non-union.

P: Most fractures will heal in by 2 months. Cord injuries cause long-term morbidity (overall 80% 10-year survival with worse survival rates in complete lesions).

D: Injury causing disruption of the bones of the wrist. Common fractures are:
Colles' fracture: Fracture of the radius within 2.5 cm of the wrist with the distal fragment becoming dorsally displaced and angulated. Often associated with an avulsion of the ulna styloid process. Originally defined in osteoporotic bone.
Smith's fracture: Fracture of the radius within 2.5 cm of the wrist where the distal fragment is impacted and anteriorly angulated.
Scaphoid fracture: Fracture of the carpal bone, scaphoid.

A: Trauma to wrist.
Colles' and scaphoid fractures: Falling onto an outstretched hand.
Smith's fracture: Falling onto a flexed wrist.

A/R: Osteoporosis.

E: Scaphoid fractures are very common, occurring in young adults. Colles' are also common and by definition occur in older persons with osteoporosis. Smith's fracture is less common.

H: History of mechanism of trauma.
Painful wrist with loss of function.

E: In all suspected fractures of the wrist, examine range of function, peripheral pulses, sensation and neighbouring joints (e.g. elbow).
Colles' fracture: 'Dinner fork' appearance of wrist and hand (see Fig. 13).
Smith's fracture: Swelling and tenderness, may appear as a Colles'.
Scaphoid fracture: Tenderness in the 'anatomical snuffbox' (on dorsal surface), scaphoid tubercle (on palmar surface) and pain on compressing thumb longitudinally.

P: The blood supply to the proximal pole of the scaphoid comes from distal nutrient vessel; hence fracture involving the waist of the scaphoid or proximal fragment can interrupt this and the proximal fragment undergoes avascular necrosis.

I: **Radiographs:** AP and lateral views of the wrist. May be necessary to view other joints for associated fractures.
Scaphoid fracture: Special scaphoid views including oblique views are needed. May need to be repeated after several days for fracture to become visible.

M: **Conservative:** If there is no displacement of the bones and no complications. Analgesic, splint the wrist with plaster of Paris and review in fracture clinic. A scaphoid cast should be used if there is any suspicion of a scaphoid fracture (extends from elbow to knuckles).
Manipulation of Colles' fracture is necessary in displacement: performed by Bier's block or haematoma block. The wrist is manipulated with disimpaction of the distal fragment, repositioning with wrist flexion and ulnar deviation and immobilisation in a below-elbow cast. Postreduction X-rays should be performed.
Surgical: Closed reduction of the fracture under anaesthesia is indicated in Smith's fractures, grossly displaced fractures or complicated fractures (or if there is normal angulation of the articular end, which is reversed in Colles' fracture). Fixation (external or internal) may be necessary. Non-union of scaphoid fracture may be treated by a bone graft or Herbert screw placed along the fracture line. Established avascualar necrosis may require excision of the fragment, radial styloid or even wrist arthrodesis.
Physiotherapy: following healing to strengthen muscles.

C: **Short-term:** Avascular necrosis (in scaphoid fractures), nerve damage (median).
Long-term: Wrist stiffness, mal-union of bones, non-union, carpal tunnel syndrome, Sudeck's atrophy, osteoarthritis.

P: Generally good in undisplaced uncomplicated fractures.

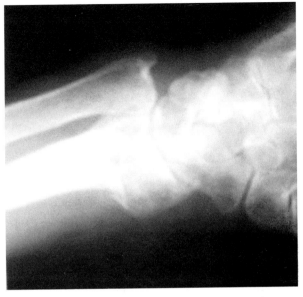

Fig. 13   Right Colles' fracture.

CONDITIONS

Gallbladder carcinoma

D: Malignancy of the gallbladder.

A: Unknown.

A/R: Strongly associated with gallstone disease (80% of patients). A 'porcelain'-bladed gallbladder (resulting from chronic cholecystitis) has an ↑ incidence of developing into malignancy. May also be associated with choledochal cysts and PSC.

E: Fifth most common GI malignancy, age usually > 65 years. Female : male is 2–3 : 1.

H: It is usually discovered incidentally on investigation for gallstone disease. The patient may present with symptoms mimicking gallstone disease, right upper quadrant abdominal pain, nausea and vomiting. Other features include weight loss, anorexia, jaundice, abdominal distension and pruritus.

E: A palpable right upper quadrant mass may be found on abdominal examination.

P: 90% are adenocarcinomas, 5% squamous carcinomas and 5% anaplastic carcinomas. They appear as gallbladder wall thickening and induration. Most common sites are in the fundus and neck of the gallbladder.
Spread: Local direct invasion into the hepatic bed, lymphatic spread into the cystic nodes, hiatal nodes, and then to the superior and posterior pancreatico-duodenal nodes and the periaortic nodes. Blood-borne spread via the portal vein to the liver.

I: **Abdominal USS:** May show gallbladder wall thickening or a mass filling the gallbladder, which would be suggestive of malignancy.
CT or MRI scan: Show a mass in the region of the gallbladder.
Arteriographic CT portogram: Where contrast is injected into the superior mesenteric artery, allows accurate assessment of the extent of the disease and its resectability.

M: **Surgical:** Simple cholecystectomy for tumours confined to the mucosa or sub-mucosa (T1a). For tumours invading the muscularis, cholecystectomy with hepatic wedge resection, resection of the cystic duct and en bloc dissection of regional lymph nodes in early-stage disease. If pericholedochal nodes are involved, the common bile duct may be resected with restoration of biliary-enteric continuity with a Roux-en-Y hepaticojejunostomy. Surgery is inappropriate for advanced disease.
Chemotherapy or radiotherapy: Some agents have partial responses (e.g. 5-fluorouracil). Radiotherapy is also used.
Palliative: Most therapy is directed at symptomatic relief. Obstructive jaundice can be managed with endoscopic or percutaneous stenting. Pain relief is a prime concern, and may be helped by percutaneous coeliac nerve block or chemical splanchnicectomy.

C: **From disease:** Obstructive jaundice, pain.
From surgery: Biliary peritonitis, haemorrhage, ascending cholangitis.

P: With the exception of cases detected incidentally at cholecystectomy, prognosis is poor as many are detected late and are not amenable to surgical resection. Overall 5-year survival of < 15%.

D: Stone formation in the gallbladder.

A: **Mixed stones:** Contain cholesterol, calcium bilirubinate, phosphate and protein (80%) due to imbalance between bile salts, phospholipids and cholesterol (supersaturation), nucleation factors and gallbladder motility.
Pure cholesterol stones (10%).
Pigment stones (10%): Black stones made of calcium bilirubinate (↑ bilirubin secondary to haemolytic disorders, cirrhosis), brown stones due to bile duct infestation by liver fluke *Clonorchis sinensis*.

A/R: **Mixed and cholesterol stones:** ↑ Age, female, obesity, DM, parenteral nutrition, drugs (OCP, octreotide), family history, ethnicity (e.g. Pima Indians), interruption of the enterohepatic recirculation of bile salts (e.g. Crohn's disease), terminal ileal resection.
Pigment stones: Haemolytic disorders (e.g. sickle cell, thalassemia, hereditary spherocytosis), residence in the Far East where liver flukes are more common. Saint's triad refers to the association of gallstones, hiatus hernia and diverticulitis.

E: Very common (UK prevalence ~ 10%), more common with age, 3× more females in younger population but equal sex ratio after 65 years. About 50 000 cholecystectomies are performed annually in the UK.

H: **Asymptomatic (90%):** found incidentally.
Biliary colic: Sudden onset, severe right upper quadrant or epigastric pain, constant in nature. May radiate to right scapula, often precipitated by a fatty meal or alcohol. It often lasts several hours, may be associated nausea and vomiting.
Acute cholecystitis: Patient systemically unwell, fever, prolonged upper abdominal pain that may be referred to the right shoulder (due to diaphragmatic irritation).
Ascending cholangitis: Classical association between right upper quadrant pain, jaundice and rigors (Charcot's triad). If combined with hypotension and confusion, it is known as Reynold's pentad.
Other complications: Obstructive jaundice, acute pancreatitis.

E: **Biliary colic:** Right upper quadrant or epigastric tenderness.
Acute cholecystitis: Tachycardia, pyrexia, right upper quadrant or epigastric tenderness. There may be guarding +/− rebound. Murphy's sign is when palpation of the right upper quadrant causes deep inspiration as the inflamed gallbladder descends and contacts the palpating fingers.
Ascending cholangitis: Pyrexia, right upper quadrant pain, jaundice.

P: Biliary colic is caused by impaction of a gallstone in the cystic duct. Resolves when stone falls back into gallbladder or stone remains impacted leading to inflammation and mucosal oedema of three histological grades: acute cholecystitis, acute suppurative cholecystitis and acute gangrenous cholecystitis. In chronic cholecystitis the pathological changes vary from microscopic evidence of chronic inflammation with the mucosa penetrating the muscle layer as Rokitansky-Aschoff sinuses to a shrunken fibrosed gallbladder with transmural fibrosis. Rarely, dystrophic calcification occurs resulting in a 'porcelain gallbladder', with ↑ risk of malignant transformation.

I: **Bloods:** FBC (↑ WBC in cholecystitis or cholangitis), LFT (↑ AlkPhos, ↑ bilirubin in ascending cholangitis. There may be ↑ transaminases), blood cultures, amylase (risk of pancreatitis).
USS: Demonstrates gallstones (acoustic shadow within the gallbladder), ↑ thickness of gallbladder wall and checks for presence of dilatation of biliary tree indicative of obstruction.

CONDITIONS

CONDITIONS

AXR: Gallstones are infrequently radio-opaque (10%) (see Fig. 14). Mainly to look for other causes of an acute abdomen.

Other imaging: Erect CXR (to exclude perforation as a differential diagnosis, ERCP, MRCP, PTC, helical CT.

M: **Conservative:** For mild symptoms of biliary colic, advice on a low fat diet may control symptoms in some patients.

Medical: Oral dissolution therapy is poorly effective, slow and has a high recurrence rate, only suitable for a small number of patients. If biliary colic is severe, this may require admission, nil by mouth, IV fluids with analgesic and antiemetics, if there are signs of infection, antibiotics should be prescribed. If symptoms fail to improve or worsen, a localised abscess or empyema should be suspected. This can be drained percutaneously by cholecystostomy and pigtail catheter. If there is ascending cholangitis, resuscitation and IV antibiotics (e.g. cefuroxime and metronidazole). If there is obstruction, urgent biliary drainage by ERCP or percutaneous route PTC.

Surgical: Laparoscopic cholecystectomy is now one of the most commonly performed operations (see Cholecystectomy, Laparoscopic).

C: **Stones within gallbladder:** Biliary colic, cholecystitis, mucocoele or gallbladder empyema, porcelain gallbladder, predisposition to gallbladder cancer (rare).

Stones outside gallbladder: Obstructive jaundice, pancreatitis, ascending cholangitis, perforation and pericholecystic abscess or bile peritonitis, cholecystenteric fistula, gallstone ileus (e.g. Bouveret's syndrome where gallstones cause gastric outlet obstruction), cholecystocholedochal fistula (Mirrizi syndrome).

Of cholecystectomy: Bleeding, infection, bile leak, bile duct damage (0.3% laparoscopic, 0.2% open), postcholecystectomy syndrome (persistant dyspeptic symptoms), port-site hernias.

P: In most cases gallstones are benign and do not cause significant problems (2% with gallstones develop symptoms annually). If they become symptomatic, surgery offers an excellent chance of cure.

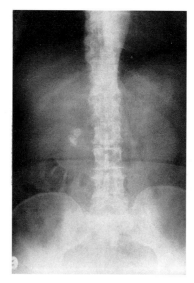

Fig. 14 Gallstones.

D: Gangrene is tissue necrosis, either wet with superimposed infection, dry (with dessication) or gas gangrene.
Necrotising fasciitis is a life-threatening infection that spreads rapidly along fascial planes.

A: Gangrene: Tissue ischaemia and infarction, physical trauma, thermal injury, inadvertent arterial injection, e.g. thiopentone and infection. Gas gangrene is caused by *Clostridia perfringens*.
Necrotising fasciitis: Typically polymicrobial with streptococci, staphylococci, bacteroides and coliforms or clostridial forms.

A/R: Diabetes, peripheral vascular disease and leg ulcers, malignancy, immunosupression and steroid use are risk factors. Necrotising fasciitis occasionally occurs without obvious predisposing factor or in relation to puncture wounds, ulcers or surgical wounds.

E: Gangrene is relatively common but gas gangrene and necrotising fasciitis are rare.

H: Gangrene: Pain with discoloration in the affected area, often the extremities or areas subject to pressure.
Necrotising fasciitis: Pain, often severe and out of proportion to the apparent physical signs.
History of risk factors or predisposing event (e.g. trauma, ulcer, surgery).

E: Gangrene: The painful area is usually the erythematous region around the gangrenous tissue, with the latter black because of haemoglobin breakdown products, dead and insensate. The junction between the live and dead tissue is known as the line of demarcation. In **wet gangrene**, the tissue becomes boggy and there may be associated pus, with a strong odour caused by anaerobes. In **gas gangrene**, spreading infection and destruction of tissues and muscle causes overlying oedema, discoloration and crepitus due to gas formation by the infection.
Necrotising fasciitis: Area of erythema and oedema, areas of haemorrhagic blisters may be present with crepitus on palpation. Associated signs of systemic inflammatory response and sepsis: temperature $> 38°C$ or $< 36°C$, tachycardia, tachypnoea, hypotension.

P: Gangrene: Tissue damage and ischaemia predispose to colonisation and proliferation of bacteria. In the presence of an anaerobic environment, synergy between organisms occurs perpetuating the cycle of tissue damage and bacterial growth. *C. perfringens*, *C. novyi* and *C. septicum* are gram-positive rod-shaped spore-forming saprophytes. They grow in the anaerobic environment of damaged tissue and produce exotoxins, e.g. α-lethicinase, which destroy the local microcirculation, cause necrosis, haemolysis and sepsis.
Necrotising fasciitis: Most commonly a synergistic polymicrobial infection spreading along the SC and deep fascial planes. Often caused by Group A β-haemolytic *Streptococcus pyogenes*, or gram-negative and anaerobic synergistic infection, e.g. enterococci, bacteroides.
Fournier's gangrene: Necrotising fasciitis of the perineum.

I: Bloods: FBC, U&Es, glucose, CRP, blood culture.
Wound swab, pus/fluid aspirate: Microscopy, Gram stain, culture and sensitivity.
X-ray of affected area: May show gas in the tissues formed by organisms.

CONDITIONS

CONDITIONS

M: **Gangrene:** Fluid resuscitation, broad-spectrum IV antibiotics with prompt surgical debridement of all necrotic tissues.

Necrotising fasciitis: Aggresive debridement of all infected tissues is necessary to limit spread and systemic sepsis together with broad-spectrum antibiotics (e.g. penicillin, aminoglycoside and metronidazole). Frequent review of the wound is necessary as the need for repeated debridement is not uncommon.

Amputation: Indicated if the limb is not salvageable or gangrene is rapidly progressive.

C: Tissue destruction, limb loss, systemic inflammatory response syndrome, sepsis, septic shock and multiple organ dysfunction syndrome.

P: Variable. If gangrenous limb is amputated early, recovery is good. Diabetes and poor peripheral vasculature are poor prognostic indicators. Gas gangrene and necrotising fasciitis are associated with high morbidity and mortality.

I: **Elective:** Tumours (benign and malignant), severe peptic ulcer disease.

A: The entrance into the stomach is via the cardiac orifice at the lower end of the oesophagus and is situated at the level of the 10th thoracic vertebra. The exit of the stomach is the pylorus leading into the duodenum; the pylorus normally lies at the level of the upper border of the 1st lumbar vertebra. The stomach can be divided into the cardia, fundus, body, antrum and pylorus, and has lesser and greater curvatures.

Vascular: The arteries supplying the stomach are the left gastric artery (from coeliac trunk), the right gastric artery (usually from hepatic artery), gastroepiploic and short gastric arteries. All of these are branches of the coeliac axis. Venous drainage is into corresponding veins that drain into the portal vein. The gastro-oesophageal junction is a site of portal–systemic anastomosis.

Lymphatics: Lymph nodes are numerous, accompany the arteries and lead to gastric, gastroepiploic, coeliac, porta-hepatic, splenic, suprapancreatic, pancreaticoduodenal, para-oesophageal, and para-aortic lymph nodes.

Nerve supply: Parasympathetic: Terminal branches of the right and left vagus nerves. Sympathetic: T6–T9 segments passing through the coeliac plexus and distributed through the greater splanchnic nerve.

I: **Imaging: AXR and CXR (erect):** In an emergency if perforation is suspected.
CT or MRI scan: For staging and assessing local resectibility.
Pre-op: Appropriate bloods: FBC, U&Es, clotting and crossmatch. In gastric tumours, a staging laparoscopy may be performed prior to definitive operation to assess resectibility.
Post-op: NG or nasojejunal tube, urinary catheter, IV fluids. DVT prophylaxis. Parenteral nutrition may be necessary in the immediate post-op period.

P: Partial gastrectomies are usually performed on the distal stomach and are referred to as Billroth (Type I or II) partial gastrectomies. Other operations are total gastrectomy, radical gastrectomy with removal of N_1 and N_2 nodes (see Gastric cancer) or an Ivor–Lewis operation for tumours of the gastro-oesophageal junction.

Incision: Upper midline or paramedian incision.
Mobilisation: Inspection is carried out with identification of anatomy. Mobilisation of the stomach with careful identification of the arteries. On the lesser curvature, the right gastric artery is ligated. On the greater curvature, the right gastroepiploic artery is ligated near the pylorus and the left gastroepiploic artery at the cardia. The duodenum is also mobilised by dividing the peritoneal attachments on the lateral border (kocherisation of the duodenum).
Partial or distal gastrectomy: The duodenum is divided between the clamps. The stomach is lifted to reveal its inferior surface. The left gastric artery is ligated. The stomach is then clamped and divided with adequate margin from the ulcer or tumour.
Reconstruction: Three different routes (see Fig. 15):
Billroth Type I: After dividing the stomach between clamps, the stomach is closed partially from the lesser curvature. The remaining unclosed portion of the stomach to the greater curvature is re-anastomosed to the duodenum.
Billroth Type II (Polya's operation): After division, the proximal gastric remnant is anastomosed to the jejunum forming a gastrojejunostomy. The proximal end of the duodenum is oversewn creating a blind loop.
Roux-en-Y: Following resection of the distal stomach, the jejunum is divided with the distal end being anastomosed to the gastric remnant, and the proximal jejunum being anastomosed to part of the distal jejunum.

C: Leakage of anastomosis, peritonitis, persistent ileus.
Long-term: Deficiency of vitamin B_{12}, early and late dumping syndromes, chronic diarrhoea, blind loop syndrome, anaemia, metabolic bone disease.

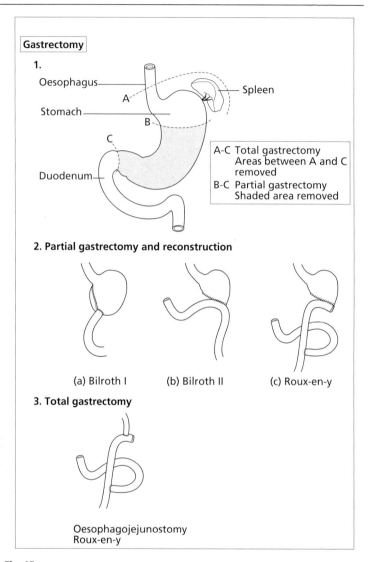

Gastrectomy

1.

Oesophagus
Stomach
A
B
C
Duodenum
Spleen

A-C Total gastrectomy
Areas between A and C
removed
B-C Partial gastrectomy
Shaded area removed

2. Partial gastrectomy and reconstruction

(a) Bilroth I   (b) Bilroth II   (c) Roux-en-y

3. Total gastrectomy

Oesophagojejunostomy
Roux-en-y

Fig. 15

D: Gastric malignancy, most commonly adenocarcinoma, more rarely lymphoma, leiomyosarcoma or stromal tumours (GIST).

A: Unknown; however, it is likely that environmental insults in a genetically pre-disposed individual lead to mutation and subsequent unregulated cell growth.

A/R: Diet high in smoked and processed foods, nitrosamines, smoking, alcohol. *Helicobacter pylori* infection and atrophic gastritis. Blood group A (1.2× relative risk). Pernicious anaemia. Partial gastrectomy. Gastric polyps. MALT lymphomas are very strongly causally associated with *H. pylori* infection.

E: Common cause of cancer death worldwide, with highest incidence in Asia, especially Japan. Sixth commonest cancer in the UK (incidence is 15/100 000). Male:female is ~2:1. Usual age of presentation >50 years. Cancer of the antrum/body is becoming less common, while that of the cardia and gastro-oesophageal junction is increasing.

H: Early often asymptomatic.
Early satiety or epigastric discomfort.
Weight loss, anorexia, nausea and vomiting.
Haematemesis, melaena, symptoms of anaemia.
Dysphagia (tumours of the cardia).
Symptoms of metastases, particularly abdominal swelling (ascites) or jaundice (liver involvement).

E: Epigastric mass. Abdominal tenderness. Ascites.
Signs of anaemia.
Eponymous signs found in metastatic spread:
Virchow's node or Troisier's sign: Palpable lymph node(s) in the left supra-clavicular fossa.
Sister Mary Joseph's node: Metastatic nodule on umbilicus.
Krukenberg's tumour: Ovarian metastases.

P: **Micro:** Adenocarcinoma, intestinal cell or diffuse subtypes (Lauren classification).
Macro: Polypoid, ulcerating (see Fig. 16) or infiltrative (Borrmann's classification), if widespread may cause *linitis plastica* (leatherbottle stomach). Gastric carcinomas can spread directly through stomach wall, via lymph nodes, trans-coelomic with peritoneal deposits or haematogenous to liver, lungs, brain, ovaries.
Staging: TNM system or the Birmingham Staging System based on clinico-pathological data.

I: **Upper GI endoscopy:** With multiquadrant biopsy of all gastric ulcers.
Bloods: FBC (for anaemia), LFT.
CT/MRI: Staging of tumour and planning for surgery.
Bone scan: Staging of tumour.
Endoscopic USS: Assess depth of gastric invasion and local lymph node involvement.
Laparoscopy may be needed to determine if tumour is resectable.

M: **Surgery:** Various surgical techniques, depending on size and location. Lymph nodes are classified in relation to the primary tumour, with those within 3 cm classified as N_1 nodes, and N_2 the second tier of nodes (removable by resection). Surgical resection is described as D1 if N_1 nodes are removed and D2 if both N_1 and N_2 nodes removed. Data from Japan has showed ↑ survival in D2 gastrectomies. Gastrectomies can be partial or total, D1 or D2 (see Gastrectomies).

Billroth I partial gastrectomy: Excision of tumour and distal stomach. Duodenal stump is anastomosed with remainder of stomach (see Fig. 15). Suitable for antral tumours.

Billroth II partial gastrectomy: Excision of tumour and distal stomach. Duodenal stump is oversewn and remainder of the stomach is anastomosed to jejunum (gastrojejunostomy) (see Fig. 15). Suitable for antral tumours.

Total gastrectomy: Removal of stomach with oesophagojejunostomy (see Fig. 15).

Ivor–Lewis gastrectomy: Proximal gastrectomy and distal oesophagectomy, with oesophago-antrostomy and pyloroplasty. Suitable for tumours of the cardia or fundus.

Palliative: Debulking surgery, gastrojejunostomy or intubation to bypass and maintain enteral nutrition.

Medical: Chemotherapy (e.g. 5-fluorouracil, platinum agents) prolongs survival by a few months. Treatment of MALT lymphomas should include eradication of *H. pylori* infection.

C: Dysphagia, gastric outlet obstruction, upper GI haemorrhage, iron deficiency anaemia. Early and late complications of gastrectomy (e.g. dumping syndrome, diarrhoea, deficiencies of B_{12}).

P: Generally poor with < 10% overall 5-year survival. About 50% in those with early disease undergoing resection.

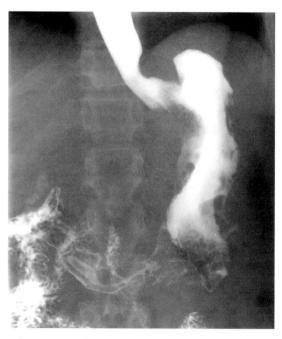

Fig. 16   Stomach carcinoma: ulcerative, with filling defects.

D: Bleeding within the GI tract.

A: **Upper GI:** *Acute or chronic*: Gastric and duodenal ulcer (50% of cases), acute erosive gastritis, oesophagitis or duodenitis, oesophageal or gastric varices, Mallory–Weiss tear, gastric angiodysplasia or Dieulafoy's malformation, tumours (uncommon).
Lower GI: *Acute*: Upper GI bleeding, diverticulitis, angiodysplasia, colitis (inflammatory, ulcerative, infective, ischaemic), colonic polyps or carcinoma. More rarely, Meckel's diverticulum, small bowel tumours, aortoenteric fistula. *Chronic*: Haemorrhoids, anal fissure, IBD.

A/R: *H. pylori*, NSAIDs and steroids are risk factors for the development or exacerbation of ulcers and erosions. Stress (Curling's ulcers) secondary to shock and ↓ splanchnic perfusion. Alcoholic binges can precipitate gastric erosions. Repeated violent vomiting ↑ the risk of a Mallory–Weiss tear.

E: A common presenting complaint or emergency presentation. 50–80/100 000 upper GI bleeds annually in the UK. More common in older individuals.

H: Haematemesis of fresh blood or dark, partly digested blood ('coffee grounds') indicating oesophageal, gastric or duodenal bleeding.
Melaena (loose black tarry offensive stools) suggests a bleed of > 50 ml occurring proximal to the caecum.
Bloody diarrhoea or fresh bleeding implies a bleed distal to the caecum.
History suggestive of cause (e.g. alcoholism, NSAID use, vomiting).

E: Features of iron deficiency anaemia (chronic GI haemorrhage).
Signs of shock (e.g. hypotension, tachycardia). Signs suggestive of aetiology.

P: See **A**.

I: **Bloods:** FBC, U&Es, clotting, LFT, crossmatch.
Oesophagogastro-duodenoscopy: Identifies site of bleeding for upper GI bleeds and allows treatment.
Sigmoidoscopy/colonoscopy: Visualises and allows treatment of colonic lesions.
Mesenteric angiography: Localises source of bleeding, but rates must be 1–1.5 ml/min to demonstrate site.
Radiolabelled RBC scan: Used to localise source if active bleeding.
Technetium scan: For ectopic gastric mucosa in Meckel's diverticulum.
Barium meal/enema: Performed once there is no active bleeding.
Laparotomy and enteroscopy: Examination of whole colon and small bowel for lesions externally and internally via a colonoscope passed through the bowel wall.

M: **Resuscitation:** Adequate IV access, active resuscitation and correction of coagulopathies.
Medical: PPI or H_2-antagonist to reduce acid secretions for ulcers. Vasopressin or somatostatin analogues (e.g. octreotide) reduce splanchnic blood flow and portal pressure and is useful in managing variceal bleeding.
Endoscopic: Upper GI endoscopy for definitive diagnosis +/− management of upper GI bleeds. Adrenaline or sclerosant injection, photocoagulation or diathermy for bleeding ulcers. Varices are treated by band ligation or injection sclerotherapy. Lower GI endoscopy may also treat source, e.g. laser photocoagulation of angiodysplasia.

CONDITIONS

CONDITIONS

Surgical: For severe bleeding or for patients who do not respond to initial endoscopic treatment, depending on site and cause, e.g. oversew of duodenal ulcer with omental patch, partial gastrectomy in upper GI bleeds or colectomy in lower GI bleeds.

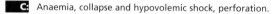 **C:** Anaemia, collapse and hypovolemic shock, perforation.

P: Depends on cause; if severe GI bleeds, aggressive resuscitation and early intervention improve outcome.

D: Perforation of the wall of the GI tract with spillage of bowel contents.

A: **Large bowel:** *Most common*: Diverticulitis and colorectal carcinoma (80%), a perforated appendix is a common complication of appendicitis. *Others*: Volvulus, ulcerative colitis (toxic megacolon), trauma, radiation enteritis and complications of post-op anastomotic dehiscence or colonosopy.
Gastroduodenal: *Most common*: Perforated duodenal or gastric ulcer, more rarely gastric carcinoma (1–2%).
Small bowel *(rare)*: Trauma, infection (typhoid, TB), Crohn's disease, lymphoma, vasculitis, radiaton enteritis.
Oesophagus: Boerhaave's syndrome is rupture following forcible vomiting against a closed glottis. Iatrogenic perforation rarely occurs during OGD but more commonly when dilatation of benign or malignant strictures is being carried out.

A/R: See above. **Gastroduodenal:** Use of NSAIDs, steroids. Curling's ulcer is associated with severe trauma, surgery or burns.

E: Incidence depends on cause (see **A**). Presentation with abdominal pain due to bowel perforation is, however, a relatively common and potentially life-threatening emergency.

H: Depends on the cause.
Large bowel: Presents usually with abdominal pain due to peritonitis. A ruptured AAA should be considered in those with sudden onset abdominal pain and shock.
Gastroduodenal: Sudden onset severe epigastric pain, worse on movement, then becoming generalised. In the elderly, the presentation may not be as acute. There may be a history of epigastric discomfort, or in gastric malignancy of pain, weight loss or vomiting.
Oesophageal: Severe pain following an episode of violent vomiting; endoscopic perforations are seen at the time of procedure, or pain in the neck or chest and dysphagia develops soon after.

E: Patient is unwell with signs of shock, pyrexia, pallor, dehydration.
Signs of localised or generalised peritonitis with abdominal rigidity and guarding, reduced or absent bowel sounds.
Loss of liver dullness occurs due to overlying gas.
In oesophageal perforations there may be SC emphysema or signs of a hydro- or pneumothorax.

P: Most perforations of the large bowel occur in the sigmoid colon, as this is a common site of diverticular disease and colorectal cancer. In most cases a pericolic abscess develops, followed by perforation. $\sim$ 15% of cases occur in the caecum following distal obstruction with a competent ileocaecal valve, as this is the most vulnerable part of the colon (Laplace's Law). The most frequent site of perforation of duodenal ulcers is in the anterior wall. In 80% of Boerhaave's syndrome there is a longitudinal tear in the left posterolateral wall of the distal oesophagus.

I: **Bloods:** FBC, U&Es, LFT, amylase (levels may be raised in perforations, but if > 3× normal, pancreatitis should be suspected), ABGs and clotting.
Erect CXR: May show air under diaphragm (see Fig. 17) (70% of cases in perforated peptic ulcer).
AXR: Can show abnormal gas shadows in tissues or in the bowel wall; alternatively, a lateral decubitus film can demonstrate intraperitoneal gas.
Gastrograffin swallow: For suspected oesophageal perforations. Alternatively, any coexisting pleural effusion aspirate would test positive for amylase.

CONDITIONS

CONDITIONS

M: **Resuscitation:** Vital pre-op with treatment of shock, correction of fluid and electrolyte abnormalities, IV antibiotics (cephalosporin and metronidazole), analgesic, urinary catheter and central line as required.

Conservative: Of gastroduodenal perforations is usually reserved for those who are a high anesthetic risk (ASA IV or V). Treatment includes nil by mouth, high-dose PPIs, IV fluids and antibiotics, NG tube and close monitoring.

Surgical:

Large bowel: Laparotomy: identification of site of perforation and peritoneal lavage. Resection of the involved colon, usually as part of a Hartmann's procedure, with formation of an end colostomy and closure of the distal stump or exteriorisation as a mucous fistula. A localised perforation of the right colon may allow resection and a primary anastomosis. In toxic megacolon of ulcerative colitis, a subtotal colectomy is performed with a terminal ileostomy and preservation of the rectal stump (allows future reconstruction of ileoanal pouch).

Gastroduodenal: Laparotomy and peritoneal lavage: the perforation is closed and an omental patch placed. Gastric ulcers should be biopsied (four quadrant, frozen section if possible) to examine for carcinoma. Closure is more difficult than duodenal ulcers and Billroth I partial gastrectomy with gastroduodenal anastomosis can be done. Post-op: *H. pylori* eradication if positive.

Oesophageal: Depends on pathology and time of presentation. If occurs during dilation of a malignant stricture, coverage by an expandable stent may be possible. If spontaneous and < 24 h from onset, should be treated surgically using a left thoracotomy with pleural lavage and primary repair, or oesophagectomy.

C: **Large and small bowels:** Peritonitis.

Oesophageal: Mediastinitis, shock, overwhelming sepsis and death.

P: **Gastroduodenal:** Higher morbidity and mortality in perforated gastric ulcers than duodenal; perforated gastric carcinomas have a very poor prognosis.

Large bowel: Untreated colonic perforation has a high risk of faecal peritonitis and death from septicaemia and multiorgan failure.

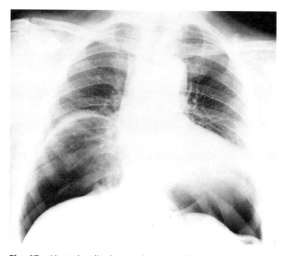

Fig. 17 Air under diaphragm: bowel perforation post surgery.

D: Inflammation of the lower oesophagus caused by reflux of gastric acid and/or bile.

A: Most common is inappropriate transient lower oesophageal sphincter relaxations and disruption of mechanisms that prevent reflux: physiological lower oesophageal sphincter, mucosal rosette, acute angle of junction (angle of His), crural fibres of the diaphragm (pinchcock mechanism), intra-abdominal portion of oesophagus, also contributing can be inefficient oesophageal antegrade peristalsis and impaired gastric motility/emptying.

A/R: Hiatus hernia, obesity, pregnancy, intake of caffeine, fat or alcohol, smoking (↑ transient lower oesophageal sphincter relaxations), drugs, e.g. tricyclic antidepressants, ↑ gastric volume (large meal, delayed gastric emptying), systemic sclerosis.

E: Common, prevalence 5–10% of adults, affecting up to 60% at some stage.

H: **Typical:** Retrosternal or epigastric discomfort, aggravated by lying supine, bending or large meals and drinking alcohol, relieved by antacids, waterbrash, regurgitation of gastric contents.
Atypical: Cardiac-type chest pain, back pain, chronic wheeze or cough, especially at night, hoarse voice, halitosis.

E: Usually normal. Occasionally, epigastric tenderness, wheeze, dysphonia.

P: Prolonged reflux of acidic stomach contents causes oesophageal mucosal inflammation, erosions and ulceration. Chronic reflux may result in a fibrotic reaction and stricture formation. Metaplasia of the lower oesophagus may occur with replacement of squamous epithelium by columnar, intestinal-type epithelium (Barrett's oesophagus) – a premalignant condition.

I: **Endoscopy:** Upper GI endoscopy, biopsy and cytological brushings to confirm the presence of oesophagitis, to grade its severity, to exclude the possibility of malignancy. Severity of reflux is graded by the modified Savary–Millar (1: erythema, 2: isolated erosions, 3: confluent erosions or superficial ulcers without stenosis, 4: erosions or deep ulceration, stricture formation).
Barium swallow: Can show structural abnormalities (e.g. hiatus hernia, stricture).
Video fluoroscopy: Can yield functional information, e.g. demonstrate reflux of contrast back into the oesophagus.
Oesophageal manometry or **24 h pH monitoring:** pH probe placed in lower oesophagus determines the temporal relationship between symptoms and oesophageal pH (significant reflux if pH < 4 for > 4.7% of time).

M: **Conservative:** Lifestyle changes, weight loss, elevating head of bed, avoid provoking factors, stopping smoking, avoiding large meals late in the evening.
Medical: Antacids or alginates, H_2 receptor antagonists, PPIs, prokinetic agents are less effective, e.g. domperidone, metoclopramide. Eradication of *H. pylori* has not been shown to improve, and is postulated to worsen GORD.
Surgical: Antireflux surgery for those with symptoms/complications despite optimal medical management or in those intolerant of medication. Open or laparoscopic fundoplication, e.g. Nissen fundoplication: after a posterior hiatal repair, the fundus of the stomach is wrapped 360° around the lower oesophagus and held with seromuscular sutures. Modifications of this method to reduce dysphagia but still prevent reflux include the Lind (270°), anterior or posterior, partial or subtotal fundoplications. Less common operations are the Hill posterior gastropexy (phreno-oesophageal bundles are sutured to the pre-aortic fascia/median arcuate ligament), in Belsey Mark IV a transthoracic approach is used to mobilise the lower oesophagus, which is then sutured to the gastric fundus.

CONDITIONS

Endoscopic: Allows for stricture dilatation. Yearly endoscopic surveillance of any Barrett's oesophagus.

C: Oesophageal ulceration, peptic stricture, Barrett's oesophagus and oesophageal adenocarcinoma.
From surgery: Persistant reflux (5–8%), dysphagia (3–8%, mostly temporary), gas bloat syndrome (difficulty belching), ↑ flatus. Rarely, oesophageal perforation, pneumothorax, splenic damage, DVT, chest infections.

P: 50% respond to lifestyle measures alone. In patients who require drug therapy, withdrawal is often associated with relapse. Antireflux surgery offers effective symptom control in 85–90% of patients.

D: Optic neuropathy with typical field defect usually associated with raised intraocular pressure (IOP).

A: **Primary:** Acute closed-angle glaucoma **(ACAG)**, primary open-angle glaucoma **(POAG)**, chronic closed-angle glaucoma.
Secondary: Trauma, uveitis, steroids, rubeosis iridis (diabetes, central retinal vein occlusion).
Congenital: Buphthalmos, other inherited ocular disorders.

A/R: **ACAG:** Hypermetropia.
POAG: Genetics, age, diabetes, myopia, race (Afro-Carribean).

E: Prevalence 1% over 40 years, 10% over 80 years (POAG), third most common cause of blindness worldwide.

H: **ACAG:** Severely painful red eye, vomiting, impaired vision, halos around lights.
POAG: Usually asymptomatic, peripheral visual field loss may be noticed.
Congenital: Buphthalmos (ox eye), watering, cloudy cornea.

E: **ACAG:** Red eye, hazy cornea, loss of red reflex, fixed and dilated pupil, eye tender and hard on palpation, cupped optic disc, visual field defect (arcuate scotoma), moderately raised IOP.
POAG: Optic disc may be cupped. Usually no symptoms.

P: Two theories for the mechanism by which elevated IOP damages nerve fibres:
(1) By causing mechanical damage to the optic nerve axons.
(2) By decreasing blood flow at the optic nerve head, causing ischaemia.
It is believed that ↑ IOP is due to ↓ outflow of aqueous humour, which can be caused by obstruction to outflow by approximation of iris to cornea, closing iridocorneal angle and trabecular meshwork/canal of Schlemm that causes a rapid and severe rise in IOP (in ACAG), resistance to outflow through trabecular meshwork (in POAG), or blockage of trabecular meshwork by blood, inflammatory cells, etc. (secondary causes).

I: **Slit-lamp examination:** See Examination.
Tonometry: To measure ocular pressure (normal 15 mmHg, POAG 22–40 mmHg, ACAG >60 mmHg).
Gonioscopy: To assess the iridocorneal angle.
Fundoscopy: To detect pathologically cupped optic disc (cup : disc is >0.6 or an asymmetry of 0.2).
Visual field testing: Arcuate scotoma (early), tunnel vision (late).

M: **ACAG (Medical emergency):** IV acetazolamide (500 mg), 4% pilocarpine topically, analgesics, antiemetics.
Long-term for POAG:
Topical: timolol (β-blockers ↓ secretion of aqueous humour).
Carbonic anhydrase inhibitor: dorzolamide (↓ secretion of aqueous humour).
Parasympathomimetics: pilocarpine (constricts pupil, opens trabecular meshwork).
Sympathomimetics: brimonidine (α_2-agonist).
Prostaglandin analogue: latanoprost (↑ flow via alternative uveoscleral drainage).
Laser treatment: Trabeculoplasty for POAG, iridotomy for ACAG.
Surgery: Drainage surgery (trabeculectomy) +/− 5-fluorouracil to prevent post-op scarring.

C: **Congenital:** Amblyopia and visual loss.
POAG: Visual loss.
ACAG: Visual loss and anterior synechiae.

P: Poor for congenital glaucoma due to amblyopia. Prognosis in acquired glaucoma depends on early diagnosis and treatment.

D: Anal vascular cushions (that contribute to anal closure) become enlarged and engorged with a tendency to protrude, bleed or prolapse into the anal canal.

A: Exact is disputed but ultimately there is disorganisation of the fibromuscular supporting stroma of the anal cushions.

A/R: Constipation, prolonged straining, derangement of the internal anal sphincter, pregnancy, portal hypertension.

E: Common (prevalence 4–5%). Peak age is 45–65 years.

H: Commonly asymptomatic.
Bleeding, usually bright red blood, on toilet paper or dripping into pan after passage of stool, can be on surface of stool but never mixed within.
Alarm symptoms should be absent (weight loss, anaemia, change in bowel habit, passage of clotted, dark blood or mucus mixed with stool).
Other symptoms are itching, anal lumps or prolapsing tissue. External haemorrhoids that have become thrombosed can cause severe pain.

E: 1st or 2nd degree haemorrhoids are not usually apparent on external inspection, and uncomplicated haemorrhoids are impalpable and only seen on proctoscopy, where they are evident as red granular mucosal swellings bulging into view on straining and withdrawal of the proctoscope at 3, 7 and 11 o'clock. Differential diagnoses include anal tags, anal fissure, rectal prolapse, polyps or tumour.

P: Excessive straining causes engorgement of the cushions, together with shearing by hard stools resulting in disruption of tissue organisation, hypertrophy and fragmentation of muscle and elastin fibres and downward displacement of the anal cushions as well as raised resting anal pressures and bleeding from presinusoidal arterioles. Classified as **internal** or **external**. Internal haemorrhoids arise from the superior haemorrhoidal plexus and lie above the dentate line while external haemorrhoids occur below the dentate line, arising from the inferior haemorrhoidal plexus. A combination of types can coexist.
Also classified by degree of prolapse:
1st degree: Haemorrhoids that do not prolapse.
2nd degree: Prolapse with defecation, but reduce spontaneously.
3rd degree: Prolapse and require manual reduction.
4th degree: Prolapse and cannot be reduced.

I: Rigid or flexible sigmoidoscopy is usually important to exclude a rectal source of bleeding as haemorrhoids are common and may coexist with colorectal tumours.

M: **Conservative:** Advice on a high-fibre diet, ↑ fluid intake, exercise, bulk laxatives. Topical creams are available that contain mild astringents combined with local anaesthetic; those with corticosteroids should only be used on a short-term basis. **Local therapy** (for 1st or 2nd degree):
Injection sclerotherapy: 5% phenol in almond oil is injected above the dentate line (no sensory fibres) into the submucosa above a haemorrhoid, inducing inflammation, with subsequent fibrosis resulting in mucosal fixation.
Banding: Barron's bands are applied just proximal to the haemorrhoid incorporating tissue that falls away after 2–3 days, leaving a small ulcer to heal by secondary intention. Higher cure rates but is more painful. Other techniques include infrared coagulation.
Surgical: Reserved for symptomatic 3rd or 4th degree haemorrhoids. Milligan–Morgan open haemorrhoidectomy involving excision of the three haemorrhoidal cushions with incisions separated by adequate skin or mucosal bridges. Stapled haemorrhoidectomy involves mucosectomy 2 cm proximal to the dentate line to 'hitch up' the prolapsing anal lining and disrupt the proximal blood

flow ($\downarrow$ pain and shorter convalescence in randomised control trials). Post-op, lactulose should be prescribed to avoid constipation.

C: Bleeding, prolapse, thrombosis and gangrene.
From injection sclerotherapy: Prostatitis, perineal sepsis, rarely impotence, retroperitoneal sepsis or hepatic abscesses.
From haemorrhoidectomy: Pain, bleeding, more rarely incontinence due to sphincteric injury, anal stricture.

P: Often a chronic problem, with recurrence of symptoms necessitating repeat local treatments. Surgery can provide long-term relief for severe symptoms.

CONDITIONS

Halux valgus

D: Foot condition where the first metatarsal bone deviates medially (metatarsus primus varus) with lateral deviation of the big toe.

A: Unknown but likely joint hypermobility in combination with biomechanical forces result in progressive deformity.

A/R: Associated family history of the condition in 50–60%. Anatomically associated with other toe deformities, e.g. hammer toe (flexion of proximal interphalangeal joint), depression of the metatarsal bones, and with a 'bunion' an adventitious bursa that forms over the prominent metatarsal head.

E: Common, often affecting adolescents and the elderly. Female > male.

H: Often asymptomatic.
Discomfort or pain due to ill-fitting shoes, an inflamed bunion, metatarsalgia or secondary osteoarthritis of the first MTP joint.

E: The patient may have a wide forefoot, with lateral deviation of the big toe.
A medial swelling or bunion is present that may be swollen and inflamed.
Skin keratoses are under the metatarsal heads.
If osteoarthritis has developed, there is ↓ range of movement in the 1st MTP joint.

P: The first metatarsal bone deviates medially (> 40° in severe cases) and also becomes dorsally angulated, with lateral displacement of the toe. Pressure of the prominent metatarsal head on overlying tissue results in synovial hypertrophy and an overlying bursa secondary to friction. Secondary osteoarthritis of the joint is common in older individuals.

I: **Radiographs (AP and lateral):** Of the weightbearing foot; the characteristic deformity is seen with medial and dorsal deviation of the metatarsal head.

M: **Conservative:** Advice to wear wider shoes. Metatarsal support cushions can help with metatarsalgia.
Mitchell's operation: An osteostomy is made through the neck of the metatarsal and the head displaced medially; performed for adolescents and young adults.
Keller's operation: In older, less active patients, the proximal third of the proximal phalanx, the medial and dorsal exostoses of the metatarsal are excised, resulting in formation of a fibrous ankylosis.
Arthrodesis of the first MTP joint: Gives good long-term function.

C: **From disease:** Pain, deformity, bursitis and synovial thickening over the MTP joint, osteoarthritis, plantar keratosis and hyperostosis.
From surgery: Recurrence of the deformity, metatarsalgia and excessive shortening of the hallux can occur with Keller's operation, stiffness of the MTP joint. Arthrodesis can be complicated by malposition, intertarsophalangeal osteoarthritis and failure of fusion.

P: Symptoms often mild, but progressive, often responding to conservative measures. Those with severe symptoms benefit from surgery; in young adults, there is a 90% success rate from reconstructive operations.

D: Primary malignancy of the liver parenchyma.

A: HCCs are associated with chronic liver damage (e.g. alcoholic liver disease, hepatitis C, autoimmune disease), metabolic disease (e.g. haemochromatosis) and aflatoxins (from cereals contaminated with fungi or biological weapons).

A/R: See **A**.

E: Common making up ∼1–2% of all malignancies, but less common than secondary liver malignancies. ↑ incidence in regions where hepatitis B and C are endemic (e.g. southern Mediterranean, Far East).

H: **History of malignancy:** Malaise, weight loss, loss of appetite.
History of exposure to carcinogens: High alcohol intake, Hepatitis B or C, aflatoxins.
Fullness in abdomen and jaundice are often the only symptoms.

E: **Signs of malignancy:** Cachexia, lymphadenopathy.
Hepatomegaly: Nodular (but may be smooth). Deep palpation may elicit tenderness.
Jaundice, ascites.
There may be bruit heard over the liver.

P: **Macro:** Grossly, HCC can undergo hemorrhage and necrosis because of a lack of fibrous stroma. Vascular invasion, particularly of the portal system, is common. Invasion of the biliary system is less common. Three common appearances: large solitary mass, multifocal nodular pattern or diffuse small foci scattered throughout the liver.
Micro: Cells resemble normal hepatocytes and can be confused with cells of hepatic adenoma. Tumours that are more differentiated can produce bile.

I: **Bloods:** FBC, ESR, LFT, clotting, α-fetoprotein, hepatitis serology.
Imaging: Abdominal ultrasound may identify a fixed lesion within a cirrhotic liver. CT scan or MRI is the gold standard for staging.
Angiography: If transarterial embolisation is being considered.
Histology: Ascites may be aspirated and sent for cytology.
Staging: Chest, abdomen and pelvic CT scans. Consider bone scan.

M: **Medical:** Chemotherapy and radiotherapy have limited role as adjuvant therapy to surgery, but may be used to control unresectable disease temporarily. Examples of chemotherapeutic agents include doxorubicin and carboplatin.
Surgical: Liver resection is indicated if localised to a single lobe. Liver transplantation can be considered if the tumour is small and the liver cirrhotic.
Embolisation: Useful for single solitary lesions in cirrhosis.
Ablation: Useful to shrink tumours not amenable to resection. Radiofrequency, cryoablation, or percutaneous ethanol injection are used.

C: Biliary tree obstruction, acute liver failure, hepatic rupture and haemoperitoneum, reactive pleural effusion, distant metastases.

P: Very poor. Majority of patients die within 1 year of diagnosis, and surgical cure is only possible in ∼5%.

CONDITIONS

CONDITIONS

D: There is a wide variety of hernias of the abdomen other than inguinal and femoral.

Incisional hernia: Herniation through a surgical incision scar.

Umbilical and paraumbilical hernia: Herniation through or around the umbilicus. Umbilical hernias occur in children, paraumbilical hernias in adults, where they usually have a narrow neck and are prone to strangulation.

Epigastric hernia: Herniation in the midline between the umbilicus and xiphisternum, through the linea alba. Associated with divarication of the rectum.

Richter's hernia: Hernias where only part of the bowel circumference is trapped within the hernial sac.

Spigelian hernia: Herniation at the lateral border of rectus abdominus, through a defect in the transverses and internal oblique fascia halfway between the umbilicus and symphysis pubis.

Obturator hernia: Herniation through the obturator foramen, producing a bulge lying below the scrotum or the labial folds.

Littre's hernia: An inguinal hernia in which the sac contains a Meckel's diverticum.

Other rare hernias include **sliding** hernias, **Maydl's** hernia (hernia-en-W), **gluteal** and **lumbar** (Petit's) hernias.

A: Weakness in the abdominal wall (e.g. due to obesity, previous surgery) and ↑ intra-abdominal pressure (e.g. coughing and straining) allows formation of the hernial sac.

A/R: Many risk factors including obesity, abdominal distension (e.g. ascites), post-op wound infection.

E: Incisional, epigastric and paraumbilical hernias are relatively common. Umbilical hernias are commonly seen in newborns, especially in Afro-Caribbeans. Other types.

H: May be asymptomatic.

Patients often notice the lump themselves. May present due to discomfort, irreducibility, ↑ in size, pain or for cosmetic reasons.

Strangulated hernias: Painful, red and swollen.

Obstruction: Constipation, colicky abdominal pain, nausea, vomiting. Richter hernias have symptoms of obstruction but still pass flatus as the bowel lumen is still patent.

E: Abdominal swelling that ↑ in size with coughing or abdominal straining.

Often nontender and soft, but may become tender and irreducible if incarcerated or strangulated. Assess for bowel sounds or signs of obstruction in acute presentation.

P: **Classification:** Hernias can be described as reducible, irreducible (incarcerated) or strangulated if there is compromise to the vascular supply of the hernia contents, e.g. omentum, bowel or abdominal organ.

I: May be diagnosed on clinical examination, or if there is any doubt about the nature of a swelling, on imaging, e.g. USS, CT scan.

In the scenario of an acute abdomen:

Imaging: AXR, erect CXR.

Bloods: FBC, U&Es, clotting, G&S, ABGs (metabolic acidosis if vascular compromise to hernia contents).

M: **Conservative:** Asymptomatic hernias with a large neck may require no treatment.

Surgical: Elective correction is indicated for umbilical hernias persisting past 2 years of age, narrow-necked hernias, irreducible hernias. The hernial sac is excised and the repair can be reinforced with a mesh. Emergency operation may be indicated in incarcerated or strangulated cases.

C: Strangulation of bowel, bowel obstruction. Epigastric hernias and obturator hernias are most likely to strangulate due to narrower necks.

P: Majority of umbilical hernias regress by 2 years of age. Other hernias usually do not regress and may progressively enlarge.

CONDITIONS

CONDITIONS

D: Prolapse of the upper stomach through the diaphragmatic oesophageal hiatus.

A: Congenital, traumatic or nontraumatic. Nontraumatic hernias can be divided into sliding, paraoesophageal (rolling) or mixed.

A/R: Obesity, low-fibre diet, chronic oesophagitis, abdominal ascites, pregnancy.

E: Common in western countries, ↑ frequency with ↑ age, from 10% in patients younger than 40 years to 70% in patients older than 70 years.

H: Majority are asymptomatic. Sliding hernias are more likely to have symptoms. If symptomatic, patients present with symptoms of GORD (i.e. heartburn, acid dyspepsia and its complications).
No correlation exists between the size of hernia and the severity of symptoms.

E: In general, there are no signs of a hiatus hernia, unless complications develop.

P: The gastro-oesophageal junction acts as an antireflux barrier. The components of this barrier include the diaphragmatic crura, the lower oesophageal sphincter baseline pressure and the angle of His. Fig. 18 shows the various types of hiatus hernias.

I: **Bloods:** FBC (for iron deficiency anaemia).
Radiology: CXR (large hernias appear as a gastric air bubble behind the heart), barium swallow or meal (allows visualisation and helps distinguish hernia types).
Endoscopy: Can be used for diagnosis of condition and complications, e.g. erosive oesophagitis, ulcers in the hiatal hernia, Barrett's oesophagus, or tumour. It also permits biopsy of abnormal or suspicious areas.

M: **Medical:** Modifying lifestyle factors (e.g. weight loss), inhibiting acid production (H_2 antagonists, PPIs), enhancing upper GI motility.
Surgical: Necessary only in the minority of patients. Indications include complications of reflux disease despite aggressive treatment, those with pulmonary complications (e.g. asthma, recurrent aspiration pneumonia). Can be done open or by laparoscopy.
Nissen fundoplication: Formation of a 360° fundic wrap around the gastro-oesophageal junction. The diaphragmatic hiatus is also repaired. A variant of the Nissen wrap and involves a 180° wrap in an attempt to ↓ the likelihood of post-op dysphagia.
Belsey Mark IV fundoplication: Involves a 270° wrap and the left and right crura of the diaphragm are approximated.
Hill repair: The cardia of the stomach is anchored to the posterior abdominal areas, e.g. the medial arcuate ligament. This augments the angle of His and strengthens the antireflux mechanism.

C: *Oesophageal complications*: May rarely be responsible for intermittent bleeding from associated oesophagitis, erosions, or a discrete oesophageal ulcer. This could lead to anaemia, Barrett's oesophagus or strictures.
Nonoesophageal complications: Incarceration of a hiatal hernia is rare and occurs only with para-oesophageal hernia. They tend to enlarge with time, and sometimes the entire stomach is found in the chest. The risk of incarceration, leading to strangulation or perforation, is ~5%. Because of the high mortality associated with strangulation, elective repair is advised for para-oesophageal hernias.

P: Generally good with most not causing severe problems (sliding hernias have a better prognosis than rolling hernias).

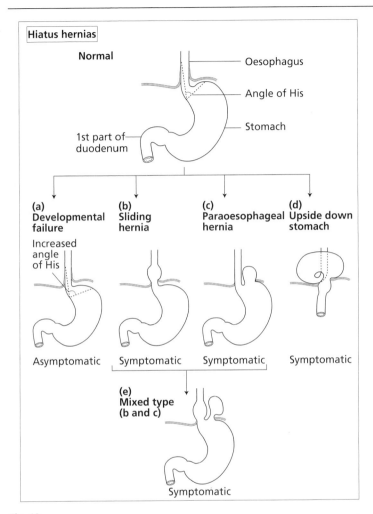

Fig. 18

Hip replacement

I: Elective: Surgical management of osteoarthritis of the hip joint and other conditions (e.g. rheumatoid arthritis, traumatic or avascular necrosis of the femoral head, sickle cell disease, congenital dysplasia). Indicated in those who have persistent pain in the hip, night pain or limited quality of life where conservative therapies (e.g. weight loss, analgesics and walking aids) are no longer effective.
Contraindications: *Absolute:* Active infection; and *Relative:* Nonambulatory patients, neurotrophic joint, abductor muscle mass loss, progressive neurological disease, skeletal immaturity, patients < 60 years are considered if other operations are unsuitable.

A: The hip joint is a multiaxial ball-and-socket synovial joint.
Relations: *Anteriorly:* Iliopsoas, pectineus, the femoral nerve and vessels. *Laterally:* Iliofemoral ligament, iliotibial tract and gluteus medius. *Posteriorly:* The gemelli, the tendon of obturator internus, quadratus femoris, the sciatic nerve and gluteus maximus. *Inferiorly:* Obturator externus.
Blood supply: From branches of the medial and lateral circumflex femoral arteries with the important retinacular vessels along the neck to the femoral head.
Nerve supply: From femoral, sciatic and obturator nerves.

I: Pre-op: Pelvis, AP and lateral hip radiographs (used to assess factors such as proximal femoral posterior bow, anterior bow at the diaphysis, medullary canal diameter) are performed in most patients. Planning of surgical approach and templating. Limb length discrepancy can be corrected through the appropriate templating of the contralateral hip and choice of prosthetic neck length. FBC, U&Es, clotting, crossmatch are minimal baseline tests. CXR and ECG, anaesthetic review.
Post-op: DVT prophylaxis; early rehabilitation; adequate analagesics.

P: Can be performed under general anaesthesia, spinal or epidural.
Approach: Most common is the posterolateral (Moore or Southern); anterolateral, transtrochanteric or anterior (Smith-Peterson) approaches are also used. Infection in a prosthetic hip is disastrous and stringent measures are used including meticulous asepsis, prophylactic antibiotics and ultraclean air operating theatres. For the posterolateral approach, the patient is positioned in the lateral decubitus position and the skin prepared and draped. After the posterolateral incision, the fascia lata is incised and gluteus maximus split and retracted to expose the posterior aspect of the hip with overlying external rotators and sciatic nerve. Using internal rotation to stretch the external rotators, stay sutures are placed into piriformis and the rotators are detached from the posterior of the greater trochanter, reflecting back to protect the sciatic nerve. The underlying joint capsule is then opened. The hip is dislocated by adduction, flexion and internal rotation. Femoral neck osteotomy is performed at the desired level. The acetabular surface is prepared and debris removed.
Choice of prosthesis: Prosthesis consists of an acetabular component made from polyethylene and the femoral component of stainless steel, titanium or cobalt chrome alloy. Components can be cemented (with methylmethacrylate that sets by an exothermic polymerisation reaction) or uncemented (whereby a porous surface allows bone ingrowth).
Minimally invasive hip arthroplasty: More recent development involving smaller incisions and less tissue trauma, thus improving recovery time.

C: Immediate: Fracture, haemorrhage, nerve injury (e.g. sciatic, femoral).
Early: DVT, infection (e.g. UTI, chest), length discrepancies, dislocation.
Late: Infection, aseptic loosening (10–20% at 10 years, but not all symptomatic), implant wear and failure, heterotopic ossification (20% at 5 years).

D: Congenital absence of myenteric ganglion cells in the rectum extending for a variable distance proximally, resulting in impaired motility and functional obstruction.

A: Failure of migration of the neural crest derived parasympathetic ganglion cell, several genes have been implicated, e.g. NCAM and RET proto-oncogene.

A/R: Familial history (5–10% cases), MEN 2A, Down's syndrome (trisomy 21).

E: Uncommon (1/5000 live births). Presents in infants or young children. Male : female is 4 : 1 in rectosigmoid disease with females tending to have longer aganglionic segments.

H: Most present under the age of 5 years.
Failure to pass meconium within 48 h of life.
Abdominal distension and vomiting.
Older children present with failure to thrive, chronic constipation, abdominal distension.

E: Abdominal distension with tinkling bowel sounds if obstruction.
PR examination may reveal a tight anal sphincter and hard stools in the rectum, and in the infant may result in sudden passage of stool and flatus, decompressing the abdomen.
May become very unwell, pyrexial with abdominal tenderness if enterocolitis develops.

P: **Macro:** 10% have short segment aganglionosis involving the terminal rectum. It involves the sigmoid colon in 75%, proximal colon in 10%, whole colon in 5%, with small bowel involvement being rare.
Micro: Histology shows characteristic lack of ganglion cells and proliferation of nerve trunks in Meissner's plexus.

I: **Imaging:** Abdominal radiographs may show multiple loops of dilated small and large bowel and an empty rectum. A barium contrast enema shows a transition zone where dilated colon becomes narrow in the aganglionic segment (see Fig. 19).
Rectal manometry: Shows absence of internal sphincter relaxation with a reduction in intraluminal pressure in the anal canal following distension of the rectum with a balloon (rarely performed except in older children).
Rectal biopsy: For definitive diagnosis, mucosal/submucosal suction biopsies without need for anaesthesia or full-thickness biopsy under anaesthesia.

M: **Surgical:** Definitive removal of the aganglionic segment is often delayed until the child is well nourished and the dilated proximal bowel has returned to normal. The bowel is deflated by defunctioning colostomy or regular rectal washouts. Alternatively, a single stage procedure without colostomy is performed in the neonatal period. Operations include Swenson, Duhamel or Soave procedures. The aganglionic segment is excised, the normal bowel pulled through and anastomosed to the anus. Presence of ganglia in the segment must be confirmed by frozen section. If present, a colostomy is closed once the anastomosis has healed.

C: Constipation, bowel obstruction, enterocolitis, caecal perforation. Of surgery: anastomotic leak with perirectal or pelvic abscess.

P: Good with appropriate management. Enterocolitis is the principle cause of mortality in untreated disease.

CONDITIONS

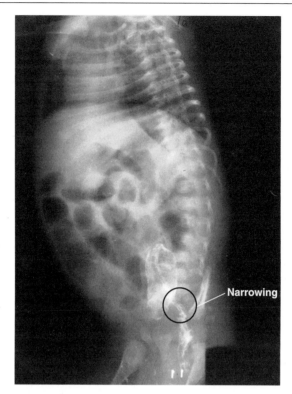

Fig. 19 Hirschsprung's disease of the rectum.

CONDITIONS

D: The excessive collection of serous fluid within the tunica vaginalis.

A: Congenital, idiopathic, tumour, infection, trauma or underlying torsion of testicle or testicular appendage.

A/R: Associated with indirect inguinal hernias in children. Epididymo-orchitis is a common cause in the UK. Filariasis is the cause of large hydrocoeles in countries of high prevalence.

E: Very common in children in their first year of life. Common in older men.

H: Scrotal swelling. Usually asymptomatic, but patient may complain of pain or urinary symptoms due to underlying cause.

E: Scrotal swelling, in which it is possible to get above the swelling, transilluminates and is difficult to feel the associated testicle as separate.

P: **Congenital:** Due to a patent processus vaginalis, the peritoneum that follows the descent of the testicle into the scrotum, with failure of obliteration leaving a small communication and peritoneal fluid tracts into the tunica vaginalis.
Idiopathic: Occurs in adults, the underlying testicle is normal and there is no apparent connection to the peritoneal cavity, i.e. noncommunicating. Contains a clear straw-coloured fluid with flecks of cholesterol. A hydrocoele of the cord (rare) is a fluid collection in part of the processus closed off to the peritoneal cavity and tunica vaginalis.
Secondary hydrocoeles: Occur acutely and develop in association with underlying inflammation of the testis or epididymis, due to infection or tumour. They tend to be smaller with the testis being palpable.

I: **USS:** To exclude underlying tumour.
Urine: Dipstick, MSU for infection.
Blood: Markers of testicular tumours if suspected (αFP, ß-HCG).

M: **Surgical:** In infants, most are resorbed spontaneously and ligation of the patent processus at the deep ring is only conducted after 1 year of age, often in association with repair of inguinal hernia. In adults, aspiration of the hydrocoele is not recommended as it tends to reaccumulate, may introduce infection or cause a haematocoele. In the younger patients, idiopathic hydrocoeles may be treated by a Jaboulay procedure whereby the tunica vaginalis is opened and the sac everted or Lord's procedure in which the sac is plicated. Secondary hydrocoeles require treatment of the underlying cause.

C: Discomfort, scrotal swelling.

P: Idiopathic hydrocoeles tend to be chronic with recurrence rates < 1% following surgical treatment. Acute secondary hydrocoeles generally resolve once the predisposing factor has been treated.

Ingrowing toenail

D: Lateral edge of a toenail grows into the soft tissue of the nail fold causing inflammation and infection. The formal term is onychocryptosis.

A: Poorly fitted footware (especially those with tapering front), poorly trimmed toenails, toe trauma, poor hygiene.

A/R: See above.

E: Common. More common in young adults and adolescents.

H: Pain along the margins of the toenail.
Painful swollen toe.
Important to enquire if patient is diabetic.

E: Erythema, oedema, warmth and pain are all features of inflammation.
Lateral side of the toenail is more likely to be affected than medial side.
Big toe (hallux) is most commonly affected.

P: The toenail penetrates the skin along its margin. The toenail can trigger a foreign body reaction, with superimposed bacterial or fungal infection causing inflammation. Tissue repair can result in exuberant granulation tissue formation.

I: None usually needed.
Pus swab: Culture and sensitivity if infected.
Radiograph (toe): In severe infection and in diabetics, it might be necessary to investigate for osteomyelitis.

M: **Medical:** Simple analgesia for pain and podiatry treatment. If presenting early, the foot should be regularly soaked and washed, with careful drying. Advice on wearing clean socks and wide fitting shoes, and importantly to cut toenails transversely. Antibiotics may be necessary if infected (after incision and drainage if pus is present), especially in diabetics
Minor surgery: For severe or recurrent cases. Performed under ring block local anaesthesia.
Incision and drainage: If there is a local collection of pus.
Wedge resection: The lateral part of the nail that is ingrowing together with nail bed (~25% of the nail) is removed, using phenol to destroy the nail bed. This relieves the pressure on the sides of the toe and prevents regrowth of the nail into the skin.
Zadek's operation: Involves removal of the entire nail and destruction of the entire nail bed.

C: Secondary infection of the nail and toe (usually fungal), deformity of nail bed and surrounding toe, permanent loss of nail.

P: Generally good if treated early. Recurrence occurs in up to 30%. In diabetics, there is a higher morbidity and can lead to loss of toe (or even limb).

CONDITIONS

D: The abnormal protrusion of a peritoneal sac through a weakness of the abdominal wall in the inguinal region.
Direct: Protrusion of the hernial sac occurring directly through the transversalis fascia and posterior wall of the inguinal canal, medial to the inferior epigastric vessels.
Indirect: Protrusion of the hernia sac, through a deep inguinal ring with coverings of the spermatic cord, following the path of the inguinal canal.

A: **Congenital:** Abdominal contents enter the inguinal canal through a persistent processus vaginalis.
Acquired: ↑ Intra-abdominal pressure together with muscle and transversalis fascia weakness.

A/R: Male, prematurity, age, obesity, raised intra-abdominal pressure, e.g. chronic cough, constipation, bladder outflow obstruction, intraperitoneal fluid, e.g. ascites.

E: Common. Congenital indirect inguinal hernias in 4% of male births. In adults peak age is 55–85 years. Men:women is 9:1. 10 elective repairs per 10 000 population carried out in the UK each year.

H: Asymptomatic or patient often notices a lump or swelling in the groin.
May present due to discomfort or pain, irreducibility, ↑ in size or symptoms of complications.

E: Groin lump that may extend to the scrotum or labia in women. Distinguished from femoral hernias by emerging above and medial to the pubic tubercle.
Examine the patient standing; the hernia is associated with a cough impulse.
Indirect hernias may be controlled by pressure over the deep inguinal ring.
Auscultation may reveal bowel sounds from within the hernia.
The hernia may be irreducible if incarcerated, very tender if strangulated, and may be associated with signs of complications, e.g. bowel obstruction and systemic upset, pyrexia and tachycardia.

P: **Classification:** Indirect (60%), direct (35%) and a combination 'pantaloon' hernia (5%). In indirect, right side is more common than left due to right testis descending later. Direct hernias emerge through Hesselbach's triangle (medially the lateral border of the rectus, laterally the inferior epigastric vessels and inferiorly the inguinal ligament). Hernias can be described as reducible, irreducible (incarcerated) or strangulated.

I: If acute with painful irreducible hernia:
Bloods: FBC, U&Es, CRP clotting and G&S if operative intervention likely. ABGs may be useful for indicating the presence of bowel ischaemia within the hernia (metabolic acidosis, ↑ lactate).
Imaging: Erect CXR and AXR (see Fig. 20), USS: May be useful in excluding other causes of groin lumps (e.g. hydrocoele).

M: **Surgical:** Elective repair for uncomplicated hernias. Can be carried out under local, epidural, spinal or general anaesthesia. There are several types of surgical repair (herniorrhaphy).
Mesh (Lichtenstein) repair: Oblique incision above the inguinal ligament, with opening of the external oblique aponeurosis and the spermatic cord gently freed. An indirect sac is dissected from the cord, opened (herniotomy) and the contents reduced. The sac is excised and the defect repaired, using a mesh to reinforce the defect in transversalis fascia. This is the most common procedure. Other open techniques include the Shouldice repair, which uses nonabsorbable sutures to reinforce the defect, and the Stoppa repair.

CONDITIONS

Laparoscopic mesh repairs: Now common with transabdominal preperitoneal and totally extraperitoneal approaches used. In general, laparoscopic repair results in earlier recovery and return to normal activities.

Emergency: Necessary in obstructed or strangulated hernia. Laparotomy with bowel resection may be indicated if gangrenous bowel is present within the hernia. Insertion of mesh may not be suitable in this case.

C: Incarceration, strangulation, bowel obstruction, Maydl's hernia (strangulated W-shaped small bowel loop), Richter's hernia (strangulation of only part of the bowel wall circumference).

From surgery: Pain, wound infection, haematoma, penile or scrotal oedema, nerve damage or neuroma formation, osteitis pubis, mesh infection, testicular ischaemia, recurrence.

P: Tend to slowly enlarge if left alone. Annual risk of strangulation 0.3–3%. Surgical mesh repair usually has a good outcome with recurrence in <5% of cases.

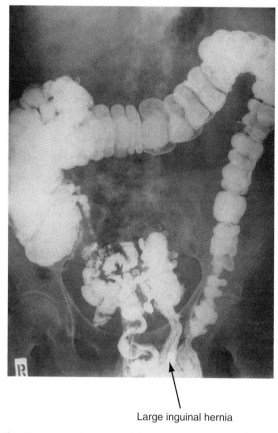

Large inguinal hernia

Fig. 20 Inguinal hernia containing both small and large bowels.

D: Obstruction (e.g. by embolus or thrombosis) of a mesenteric vessel leading to bowel ischaemia and necrosis.

A: Embolus (60%), arterial thrombosis (25%), venous thrombosis (15%). May be a consequence of volvulus, intussusception, bowel strangulation within a hernia, or failed surgical resection.

A/R: Atrial fibrillation, mural thrombus and endocarditis for emboli. Hypercholesterolaemia, hypertension, DM and smoking for arterial thrombosis.
Venous thrombosis is associated with portal hypertension, splenectomy, septic thrombophlebitis, external compression of the superior mesenteric vessels and cardiac failure. The risk of venous thrombosis is ↑ in users of OCP and in persons with thrombophilic conditions.

E: Uncommon. More common in older individuals.

P: Occlusion of mesenteric vessels results in acute bowel ischaemia, progressing to infarction if not relieved, with oedema and haemorrhage into the bowel wall, lumen and peritoneal cavity. Gangrene and bowel perforation commonly develop.

H: Severe acute colicky abdominal pain.
May be associated with vomiting or rectal bleeding.
History of chronic mesenteric artery insufficiency (e.g. gross weight loss and abdominal pain following eating).
History of heart or liver disease.

E: Diffuse abdominal tenderness and abdominal distension.
A tender palpable mass (the ischaemic bowel) may be found (especially if associated with hernia).
Bowel sounds may be absent.
Disproportionate degree of cardiovascular collapse.

I: Diagnosis is difficult, may be based on clinical suspicion or found at laparotomy.
AXR: May show thickening of small bowel folds and gas appearing within the bowel wall (late signs).
Bloods: ABG (lactic acidosis), FBC, U&Es, LFT, clotting, crossmatch.
Mesenteric arteriography: If stable, allows localisation, a measure of the extent of involvement and a trial of intervention.

M: **General:** Nil by mouth, IV fluid resuscitation and correction of electrolyte imbalances, general anaesthetic review.
Surgical: Emergency laparotomy and resection of infarcted bowel. Arterial supply to non-necrotic bowel may be restored by embolectomy or by using a saphenous vein bypass from the iliac artery to the superior mesenteric artery below the obstruction. A temporary defunctioning stoma is often used. Close monitoring and care is required post-op, usually on HDU or ITU. Rarely, extensive small bowel resection has been supported by total parenteral nutrition followed at a later stage by small bowel transplantation.
Medical: Thrombosis prophylaxis with heparin post-op is essential. Long-term warfarinisation may be indicated.

C: Lactic acidosis, bowel perforation, peritonitis, multi-organ dysfunction.

P: A serious condition that has a high mortality (50–100%).

Intestinal obstruction

D: Obstruction of the normal movement of bowel contents. Classified according to site: small or large bowel, partial or complete, simple or strangulated.

A: **Extramural:** Hernia, adhesions, bands, volvulous.
Intramural: Tumours, inflammatory strictures, e.g. in Crohn's disease or diverticulitis, intussusception.
Intraluminal: Pedunculated tumours, foreign body, e.g. bezoars, gallstones; infection, e.g. worms.

A/R: See **A**.

E: Common. More common in elderly due to increasing incidence of adhesions, hernias and malignancy.

H: Severe gripping colicky pain with periods of ease, located in the central (small intestine) or lower abdomen (large intestine).
Abdominal distension.
Frequent vomiting of greenish bile-stained vomit, early in SBO or late with faeculent vomiting in distal SBO or LBO.
Absolute constipation – failure to pass either stool or flatus.

E: Abdominal distension with generalised tenderness. Visible peristalsis may be seen.
↑ Bowel sounds ('tinkling' in character). Guarding and rebound suggest peritonitis has developed, bowel sounds may be absent.
Inspect for hernias. Multiple abdominal scars suggest adhesions.
Inspect for abdominal mass (e.g. in intussusception, carcinoma, mass in the pouch of Douglas, faecal impaction).

P: **Simple obstruction** (bowel occlusion without vascular compromise)**:** Intestine distal to occlusion rapidly empties and collapses while bowel above the obstruction dilates with gas and fluid. With ↑ distension, the intestinal wall blood supply becomes impaired and mucosal ulceration and bowel perforation may occur.
Strangulated obstruction: The blood supply to the affected segment is severed leading to impairment of the normal mucosal barrier with bacterial transudation into the peritoneal cavity and peritonitis, with the unrelieved bowel developing gangrene and perforating.

I: **AXR (erect and supine):** Assists diagnosis and localisation of obstruction. Central dilated loops with valvulae conniventes crossing the entire width of bowel suggests SBO. If distended bowel lies more peripherally, with haustrations that do cross the bowel width, this suggests LBO. Fluid levels may be seen.
Water-soluble contrast enema: In LBO, can demonstrate the site of obstruction.
Barium follow-through: Can identify strictures in SBO.

M: **General:** Gastric aspiration by NG tube if vomiting. Resuscitation with IV fluids and electrolyte replacement, close monitoring of vital signs, fluid balance, urine output and clinical status. Conservative measures may settle an acute obstruction; however, if not resolving or signs of complications, operative intervention should be carried out.
Surgical: Emergency laparotomy in acute obstruction where there is a risk of strangulation with resection of nonviable bowel and primary anastomosis in small bowel resection or Hartmann's operation or hemicolectomy with defunctioning stoma in large bowel resection. Post-op care in an HDU or ITU setting may be required.

C: Dehydration, bowel perforation, peritonitis, toxaemia, gangrene of ischaemic bowel wall.

P: Variable. Dependent on general state of patient and prevalence of complications.

D: Haemorrhage within the brain parenchyma with formation of a focal haematoma.

A: Hypertension and trauma are the most common causes. Other causes include arteriovenous malformation, intracerebral aneurysms, cavernous haemangiomas, tumours, bleeding into a previously infarcted region and drug abuse (e.g. amphetamines).

A/R: Hypertension, anticoagulation and Alzheimer's disease (amyloid angiopathy).

E: 15% of strokes. 15–300/100 000 incidence. Peak incidence in older age groups.

H: Sudden development of stroke syndrome, symptoms depending on site of haemorrhage (e.g. contralateral weakness, speech disturbance if in dominant hemisphere).
Deteriorating level of consciousness.
Headache and vomiting.

E: **Signs of stroke syndrome:** Hemiparesis, sensory loss, cranial nerve lesions, cerebellar ataxia, loss of higher cognitive functions.
Signs of ↑ ICP: ↓ GCS, ↑ BP.
Unequal pupils may indicate developing herniation.

P: Chronic hypertension is associated with the development of Charcot–Bouchard micro-aneurysms that are often the source of bleeding. Extravasation of blood compresses surrounding parenchyma. May progress outwards onto the surface of the brain (becoming a subarachnoid haemorrhage) or inwards into the ventricular system (intraventricular haemorrhage). The putamen is a common site of spontaneous intracerebral bleeds, followed by the caudate.

I: **CT or MRI brain:** Indicated for all strokes to distinguish ischaemic from haemorrhagic strokes. Features of severity include signs of raised ICP, midline shift and hydrocephalus.
Angiography: May be indicated if suspicion of underlying vascular malformation.

M: **Emergency:** Attention to ABC; intubation and ventilation may be necessary with ↓ GCS. Supportive care with resuscitation and correction of coagulation and electrolyte abnormalities.
Surgical: Evacuation of haematoma if large and ↑ ICP. Interventional radiology may be helpful in cases involving isolated aneurysms.
Treat complications: Monitoring and treatment of ↑ ICP (e.g. insertion of pressure monitoring bolt and/or external ventricular drain in hydrocephalus). Cautious use of antihypertensives (e.g. labetalol) should be considered in severe hypertension but there is a risk of watershed infarction.
Supportive: Nutritional support (NG feeding), care of pressure points, speech and language therapy, rehabilitation.

C: ↑ ICP, hydrocephalus (especially in posterior fossa haemorrhage) herniation, neurological deficits.

P: High mortality, with GCS score on admission and size of haematoma being strong predictors of prognosis.

CONDITIONS

CONDITIONS

D: The process of invagination of an intestinal segment into the adjoining intestinal lumen potentially resulting in vascular compromise of the bowel or obstruction.

A: **In toddler (<3 years old):** Majority of cases are associated with lymphoid hyperplasia in Peyer's patches. In ~ 10% of cases, the lead point is a Meckel's diverticulum or a polyp.
In juvenile/adult: Mass in bowel wall or lumen (e.g. lymph node, polyp, tumour).

A/R: Associated with recent URTIs, blood dyscrasias (due to submucosal haematomas), Henoch-Schönlein purpura.

E: Incidence is 1–4/1000. Usually affects infants and toddlers < 3 years old (majority occur in 5–10-month-olds). Rare in adults.

H: A child presenting with intermittent episodes of severe abdominal pain. In younger children this is often accompanied by drawing up of legs.
Bloody mucus can be passed PR that is said to resemble 'currant jelly'.
In later stages, it can resemble bowel obstruction with vomiting and distension.

E: Classically, 'sausage-shaped' mass in right hypochondrium.
Signs of shock: Pale, hypotensive, tachycardia.
Signs of obstruction: Abdominal distension, tinkling or absent bowel sounds.
Signs of perforation: Rigid abdomen with guarding.

P: **Pathogenesis:** Believed to involve abnormal peristalsis causing a portion of the intestinal wall (intussusceptum) to invaginate into adjoining segment (intussuscipiens). The ileocolic junction is the commonest site, although ileo-ileal and colo-colic also occur.

I: **AXR:** May show absence of air on the right side of the bowel or features of SBO.
Ultrasound: Insussception appears as a doughnut on the scan.
Barium/air enema: This is the classical way of showing intussusception, with contrast at the site showing a 'coiled spring' appearance. This can be therapeutic (see **M**).
Bloods: FBC, U&Es, ABG (for lactic acidosis), G&S.

M: **Supportive:** Resuscitation with IV fluid, analgesics, antibiotic cover, NG tube insertion if vomiting.
Therapeutic enema: The intussusception may be reduced by the pressure of contrast pushing the invaginating segment (the lead-point) back. Contraindicated if there is perforation, peritonitis, or if a mass is known to be the cause.
Surgical: Performed if failure to resolve with enema or if there are signs of peritonitis. The affected bowel is gently manipulated to reduce intussusception. If the involved bowel is nonviable, cannot be reduced or Meckel's is found, resection of the involved segment is necessary.

C: Can lead to ischaemia, haemorrhage, obstruction, perforation.

P: Good with prompt treatment (mortality ≤ 1%). Recurrence rate is 1–5%.

D: Limb ischaemia due to sudden occlusion of the supplying artery.

A: **Thrombosis:** For example, in atherosclerotic vessels.
Embolism: 90% from heart, 9% from great vessels, 1% other.
Vascular injury: For example, trauma or dissection.

A/R: **T:** Atherosclerosis, aneurysm, graft stenosis, thrombotic states.
E: Atrial fibrillation, recent MI, valvular heart disease, aneurysms, atrial myxoma may also occur during interventional radiological procedures.

E: Uncommon but incidence may be increasing.

H: **6 Ps:** **p**allor, **p**ain, **p**arasthesiae, **p**ulselessness, **p**aralysis and '**p**erishingly' cold limb. Embolus more likely if severe, sudden onset and potential source identifiable (e.g. atrial fibrillation or recent MI).
Thrombosis usually if less severe (collaterals present), history of claudication or peripheral vascular disease, no obvious source of embolus.

E: Limb is pale with absent pulses, capillary return is slow.
After several hours there is venous stagnation with a resulting mottled appearance and fixed staining in late stages due to capillary rupture.
Sensation is altered and if ischaemia is severe, anaesthesia with muscle paralysis, signifying the limb may be nonviable.

P: Sudden interruption of blood supply. There are two phases of cell injury: (1) ischaemic injury as tissues are deprived of blood supply; and (2) reperfusion injury if blood flow is restored.

I: **Bloods:** FBC, U&Es, coagulation profile, G&S, thrombophilia screen.
Imaging: CXR, Doppler or duplex scanning of blood flow, arteriography to demonstrate the site of occlusion and plan intervention if limb viable.
ECG: Looking for atrial fibrillation.

M: **Immediate:** Analgesia, heparin anticoagulation to prevent thrombus propagation. Appropriate medical treatment for associated cause.
Surgical: Revascularisation within 6 h in order to salvage limb. Operative risk is often high due to underlying heart disease.
If embolus: Embolectomy, which involves isolation of artery, arteriotomy and introduction of a Fogarty balloon-tipped catheter that is passed beyond the embolus, the balloon inflated and withdrawn to retrieve the embolus.
If acute or chronic thrombosis: The limb may remain viable for longer due to collateral formation and intra-arterial thrombolysis is an option, with local infusion of, e.g. t-PA, with angioplasty of underlying stenoses.
If thrombosis but the limb is not likely to remain viable for the 12–24 h necessary for this procedure: Urgent reconstructive surgery is required, if technically possible with autogenous (saphenous vein) or synthetic (e.g. PTFE or Dacron) bypass grafting. Under some circumstances, fasciotomy is required.
If nonviable limb: Limb amputation is required.

C: **From disease:** Gangrene, limb loss, death.
From intra-arterial thrombolysis: Mortality (1–2%), CVA, major haemorrhage.
Post-treatment: Reperfusion syndrome, compartment syndrome.

P: Only 60–70% are discharged with an intact limb, a major mortality factor is underlying cardiac disease.

CONDITIONS

D: Chronic arterial insufficiency to the lower limbs resulting in consequences ranging from pain on exercise (intermittent claudication) to ulceration or gangrene.

A: Atherosclerosis in the lower aorta, iliac, femoral or other leg arteries.

A/R: Smoking, hypertension, diabetes, hypercholesterolaemia, family history.

E: Common, prevalence 7–15% of elderly population, male:female is 2:1. Annual incidence of critical limb ischaemia is 50–100/100 000 in the UK.

H: **La Fontaine** classification system of symptoms:
I: Asymptomatic.
II: Intermittent claudication. Crampy pain in the calf, coming on during exercise after a constant distance (claudication distance), relieved within a few minutes of exercise cessation.
III: Rest pain. Severe aching pain that typically comes on in the lower limb at night, with some relief by hanging the leg over side of bed.
IV: Limb ulceration or gangrene.
Critical ischaemia: When there is rest pain > 2 weeks, ulceration or gangrene, indicating severe arterial insufficiency threatening the viability of the limb.
Leriche's syndrome: When buttock and thigh claudication and impotence result from lower aortic occlusion.

E: Examine the cardiovascular system, looking for signs of hyperlipidaemia, carotid bruits, signs of ischaemic heart disease, abdominal aortic aneurysm.
If ischaemia is severe in lower limbs, there is shiny atrophic skin with hair loss or atrophic nails, ulcers tend to be painful and have a 'punched out' appearance (e.g. under toes or classically over lateral malleolus). Peripheries cool to the touch with prolonged capillary return time, weak or absent pulses. Listen for bruits.
Buerger's test: Elevation of the leg results in pallor, venous guttering, followed by dependent rubor.
Ankle-brachial pressure index: Measured using a handheld Doppler; determined as the systolic ankle pressure divided by the brachial pressure. Normal > 0.9; claudication 0.8–0.6.
Critical ischaemia < 0.5 or ankle systolic < 50 mmHg or toe systolic < 30 mmHg. (Values may be falsely high in diabetics due to poorly compressible vessels, and absent pulses on palpation replace pressure measurement.)

P: Atherosclerosis causes stenoses in the arterial tree; at rest there must be a > 80% area narrowing before there is a fall in perfusion pressure. During exercise, demand is ↑ and inadequate oxygenation results in relative ischaemia and pain. Critical limb ischaemia is usually due to multisegment disease causing severe ischaemia, such that tissue viability is threatened with risk of ulceration and gangrene.

I: **Imaging:** Colour duplex may localise disease; however, the gold standard is still angiography, usually digital subtraction angiography as this uses smaller doses of contrast. This should only be performed on those in whom intervention is likely. Use of MRA is increasing (no risk of ionising radiation).
Bloods: FBC (for polycythaemia or thrombocythaemia), lipid (for hyperlipidaemia), random glucose (for diabetes).

M: **Medical:** Stop smoking and exercise, supervised programs have been shown to be effective. Treatment of other cardiovascular risk markers, e.g. statins, control of hypertension (but β-blockers should be avoided as they tend to ↓ peripheral circulation), aspirin. Prostacyclin infusions are sometimes used in those with critical ischaemia unable to tolerate other interventions but this can cause severe hypotension.

Endovascular techniques: Percutaneous transluminal angioplasty is used to dilate arterial stenoses, the optimum lesions are short stenoses with good run-off. Endovascular stents are used for significant stenoses above the inguinal ligament.

Surgical: For critical ischaemia or incapacitating IC.

Revascularisation: Method depends on the site of occlusion and may be combined with endovascular techniques.

Aortoiliac occlusive disease: Aortobifemoral bypass or rarely axillobifemoral bypass, unilateral iliac disease (femoro-femoral or iliofemoral bypass).

Femoropopliteal disease: Femoropopliteal, femorotibial or femorodistal bypass grafting using autogenous, e.g. saphenous vein (either reversed or in situ with valves destroyed with valvulotome) or synthetic grafts, e.g. PTFE. With the latter, a vein patch (Millar cuff) at the distal anastomosis significantly improves longer-term patency rates. Post-op surveillance of the graft by duplex scanning is essential.

Amputation: Indicated for end-stage atherosclerotic disease, if revascularisation is technically impossible or there is significant necrosis or spreading sepsis. Revascularisation may enable below knee amputation rather than above knee, the former associated with better post-op mobility and prosthetic limb use.

C: Pain, ulceration, gangrene if wet, risk of systemic sepsis and multiorgan dysfunction.

From angioplasty: 3–4% risk of complications, e.g. groin haematoma, acute thrombosis of the dilated segment.

From bypass grafting: *Early*: Risk of cardiac events, graft thrombosis, haemorrhage, lymphocoele, oedema, infection.

Late: Thrombosis, false/anastomotic aneurysm, graft stenosis. In general, patency rates above knee (70–80% at 3 years) > below knee, small risk graft infection.

P: Lower limb ischaemia is a marker of atherosclerosis throughout the vascular tree and patients are at ↑ risk of MI and stroke. ~40% individuals with intermittent claudication will improve, 40% will remain stable and 20% progress over 5 years requiring intervention.

CONDITIONS

Knee replacement

I: **Elective:** Painful arthritis of the knee (osteoarthritis is the most common indication).

A: The knee joint is a hinge joint articulating the femur and the tibia. The articular surface of the femur is the medial and lateral condyles. The articular surfaces are lined with the semilunar-shaped medial and lateral meniscus. Anterior to the knee joint is the patellar that articulates with the femur. The knee is supported by four ligaments: the anterior and posterior cruciate ligaments (named after the site of attachment on the tibia) and the lateral and medial collateral ligaments. The mechanical axis of the lower limb is an imaginary line through which the weight of the body passes, running from the centre of the hip to the centre of the ankle through the middle of the knee.
Surrounding muscles: Anteriorly lies the quadriceps femoris; laterally the tendons of the biceps femoris and popliteus. Medially lie the sartorius, gracilis, semitendinosus and semimembranosus.
Vascular: Arterial supply derives from the highest genicular artery, a branch of the femoral, the genicular branches of the popliteal artery, the recurrent branches of the anterior tibial artery, and the descending branch from the lateral femoral circumflex artery of the profunda femoris. Nerve supply is derived from the obturator, femoral, tibial and common peroneal nerves.

I: **Knee radiographs:** AP and lateral views are usual first-line investigations for any knee suspected of arthritis.
Pre-op: Nil by mouth, crossmatch at least 2 units, antibiotic prophylaxis. Operation should ideally be performed in an operating theatre designed for laminar flow of air to prevent contamination of prosthesis.
Post-op: Antibiotic prophylaxis, mobilise as soon as drain is removed. DVT prophylaxis is essential.

P: This operation is variable depending on the prosthesis used; as such only a general description of the procedure is given here.
Access: A thigh tourniquet is often used to reduce blood loss. Medial parapatellar incision anteriorly extending from the quadriceps muscle to the tibial tubercle running along the medial border of the patella.
Procedure: The infrapatellar fat pad is excised and the patella is flipped upwards so that the articular surface faces upwards. Soft tissues of the knee joint (i.e. meniscus, cruciate ligaments) are excised together with any osteophytes. Femoral and tibial surfaces are prepared as per the prosthesis used; this usually involves bone cuts of the femur and tibia perpendicular to the mechanical axis of the respective bones with careful measurements to ensure the loadbearing on the knees remains symmetrical. Once the prosthesis is sited, it is cemented in place with polymethylmethacrylate cement. Tourniquet is removed to assess haemostasis and knee joint is tested passively.
Closure: Capsule is closed using interrupted sutures and a drain may be left in situ. Skin closure with interrupted or subcuticular sutures.

C: Infection of prosthesis, osteomyelitis, DVT, patellofemoral subluxation and instability, damage to the popliteal artery, vein or femoral nerve.

I: Lacerations or cut penetrating the layers of the skin and underlying tissues.

A: The skin is divided into three layers:
(1) Epidermis – outer keratinised epithelium;
(2) Dermis – underlying fibroelastic layer containing blood vessels, lymphatics and nerves;
(3) SC – deep layer of variable thickness comprising mostly adipose tissue.

I: Radiograph may be necessary if there is risk of foreign body such as glass or associated bony injury.

P: Simple lacerations may be closed primarily, e.g. in an accident and emergency department. More complex injuries, especially involving face or complicated by other injuries, e.g. tendon damage, are best referred to appropriate specialists, e.g. plastic surgeons. It is always important to consider tetanus status and give booster or immunoglobulin and immunisation as appropriate. If associated with a fracture, i.e. an open fracture, antibiotics should be given. For cuts caused by bites, primary closure is avoided and antibiotics given, especially if it is a human bite.

Local anaesthesia: The wound is anaesthetised by first raising a small skin bleb of local anaesthetic using needle and syringe. Local anaesthetic is then injected more widely, ensuring aspiration prior to injection to avoid intravascular injection. Local anaesthetic mixed with adrenaline should never be injected near digits or areas such as nose, ear or penis.

Inspection and wound toilet: The wound is inspected and thoroughly irrigated and cleaned. This may require vigorous scrubbing if dirty. The wound is inspected for any underlying damage, e.g. to underlying tendons.

Type of suture: If deep tissues require suturing, SC absorbable sutures are used. Otherwise nonabsorbable sutures are always used, with width according to site, e.g. 5–0 or 6–0 fine sutures for face, 3–0 or 4–0 for trunk/arms.

Suturing: For a diagrammatic summary of types of sutures see Fig. 21. Aseptic technique should be used with appropriate wound preparation and draping. The following are the simple discontinuous (interrupted) sutures:
(1) Using a needle holder, the needle is inserted at right angles to the tissue, reaching into the depth of the wound, passing through both sides of the suture line and exiting at right angles. The distance from the entry or exit point to the edge of the wound should be roughly equal.
(2) Using a forceps, the needle and suture is pulled through to leave a long end with the needle and a short end.
(3) The long end is now looped clockwise around the needleholder and the short end is grasped by the needleholder and pulled through the loop keeping the knot to one side of the suture line.
(4) This is now repeated again but the long end of the suture is looped anticlockwise instead making sure to keep the knot on the same side of the suture line to produce a reef knot.
(5) The knot is repeated again with the loop made clockwise again to produce a standard surgical knot. The suture is cut short close to the knot.
(6) Successive sutures are placed with all sutures at right angles to the wound and equidistant apart. One way to ensure equidistance is to start suturing at the midpoint of the laceration.

Other types of sutures, e.g. mattress sutures, may be used for deeper or more complex wounds.

Dressing: A dry dressing is applied to the wound. Stitches are kept in place only as long as needed to provide support to the wound. Stitches on the face are removed within 2–5 days, whereas limb and abdominal wall stitches usually remain for 7–10 days.

C: Wound infection, poor healing or scar formation.

CONDITIONS

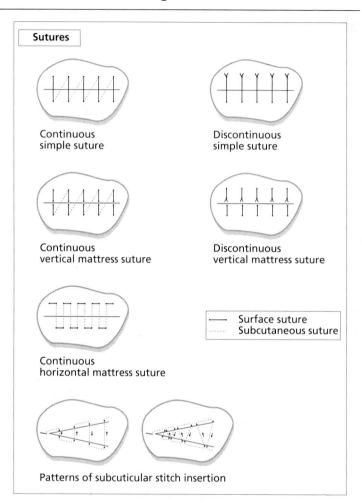

Sutures

Continuous
simple suture

Discontinuous
simple suture

Continuous
vertical mattress suture

Discontinuous
vertical mattress suture

Continuous
horizontal mattress suture

—— Surface suture
······· Subcutaneous suture

Patterns of subcuticular stitch insertion

Fig. 21 Types of sutures.

I: Minimal access surgery of the abdomen or pelvis, whereby following creation of a pneumoperitoneum, a rigid endoscope is introduced into the peritoneal cavity, through a sleeve, for inspection and to guide manipulation by other instruments introduced through other ports.

Diagnostic: Used in the investigation of abdominal or pelvic pain, focal liver disease, abdominal masses, staging of malignant disease, for directed biopsy or emergency evaluation of abdominal trauma.

Therapeutic: Abdominal operations. Most common procedure is cholecystectomy, but others include appendicectomy, fundoplication, hernia repair, splenectomy, rectopexy, nephrectomy for benign disease, palliation of incurable disease by resection or bypass. Laparoscopy can be used to assist in other procedures, e.g. laparoscopic-assisted hysterectomy.

Absolute contraindications: Active infection of the abdominal wall near entry sites.

Relative contraindications: Uncorrected coagulopathy, respiratory insufficiency, the presence of distended bowel. Obesity and previous surgery ($\uparrow$ likelihood of adhesions) may make conversion to open operations more likely.

A: Physiological consequences of a pneumoperitoneum are usually well tolerated in otherwise fit patients but may be less so by those with cardiac disease.

Cardiovascular: $\downarrow$ Cardiac output, $\uparrow$ systemic and pulmonary vascular resistance, $\uparrow$ cardiac preload, $\downarrow$ hepatic, splanchnic and renal flow.

Metabolic and autonomic: $\uparrow$ Renin and aldosterone, sympathomimetic response and renal vasoconstriction.

I: As appropriate for the intended procedure.

P: Can be performed under general or local anaesthesia.

Preparation: NG tube and urinary catheterisation can be used to decompress the stomach and bladder, respectively, depending on the intended procedure. Preparation and draping of the abdomen is performed.

Pneumoperitoneum: An initial longitudinal or transverse, infra- or supraumbilical incision is made. Can be done by an open (Hasson) or closed method:

Open: Following dissection of the initial incision, the linea alba is identified and incised. The peritoneum is identified, picked up with two clips and opened, ensuring that no bowel has been caught by the clips. A threaded cannula can be used to minimise gas leak.

Closed: The abdominal wall is manually elevated and a Veress needle is introduced into the peritoneal cavity. Controlled pressure insufflation of the peritoneal cavity with CO_2 (up to 10–12 mmHg) is then performed. $\uparrow$ Risk of damage to bowel or blood vessels due to being done blind.

Insertion of laparoscope: The laparoscope is introduced after adjustment of the white balance (to compensate for the yellow light of the halogen bulb) and used to visualise the peritoneal cavity and safely guide introduction of further ports.

Closure: Following the intended procedure, the instruments and ports are removed, allowing deflation of the pneumoperitoneum and appropriate wound closure.

C: **Immediate:** Injury to viscera or vessels, extraperitoneal insufflation, diaphragmatic splinting due to excessive insufflation. Rarely, pneumothorax or gas embolism.

Early: Shoulder tip pain, wound infection, consequences of unrecognised visceral injury (e.g. peritonitis following bowel injury or consequences of bile duct injury).

Late: Incisional hernia, port-site metastases in cases of malignancy.

Lipomas

D: Lipomas are slow-growing benign tumours of adipose tissue.
Lipomatosis refers to multiple contiguous lipomas that cause distortion of SC tissues (e.g. on buttock or rarely, neck).
Lipomas can be classified by location, e.g. SC, subfascial, subsynovial.

A: Unknown, certain chromosomal aberrations have been implicated (e.g. translocation of a gene on chromosome 12).

A/R: A rare presentation is multiple tender lipomas (Dercum's disease/*adiposis dolorosa*).

E: All ages, mostly 40–60 years, rare in children. No gender preference.

H: Patient notices a lump, usually painless and slowly enlarging, unless subject to trauma when fat necrosis may cause it to swell and become tender.

E: Can occur anywhere there are adipose tissue reserves, common in the SC tissue of the upper arms.
Nontender, soft, compressible, but do not usually fluctuate or transilluminate except if large. Lipomas do not have a fluid thrill and are dull to percussion. The overlying skin is usually normal. Variable size, usually ovoid or spherical, often lobulated (a useful diagnosic feature).
Local lymph nodes should not be palpable.

P: Can arise in any connective tissue but are most common in SC fat. Histologically, they are made up of collections of adipose cells indistinguishable from normal adipocytes divided into large lobules by thin fibrous septa.

I: Usually none necessary; MRI can be used for visualising deeply sited lipomas.

M: **Conservative:** May be left alone if not causing discomfort or distorting appearance.
Surgical: If troublesome or unsightly. Can be removed under local anaesthesia: an incision is made over the lipoma to expose it; a typical feature is that the lipoma can be milked out through the incision by gentle pressure on the surrounding tissue, often with minimal dissection. Haemostasis in the resulting cavity should be ensured to avoid haematoma development. Larger lipomas or those in more complicated sites will need excision under general anaesthetic.

C: If traumatised, may undergo fat necrosis.

P: Excellent; as a general rule, lipomas do not become malignant (liposarcomas usually arise *de novo*, e.g. in the retroperitoneum).

D: Infection resulting in a walled-off collection of pus in the liver.

A: **Pyogenic:** *Escherichia coli, Klebsiellae, Enterococci, Bacteroides, Streptococci, Staphylococci.*
Amoebic: *Entamoeba histolytica.*
Hydatid cyst: Tapeworm, *Echinococcus granulosis.*

A/R: **Pyogenic:** 60% due to biliary tract disease (e.g. strictures), cryptogenic (15%).
Amoebic/hydatid: Foreign travel.

E: **Pyogenic:** Annual incidence is 0.8/100 000. Mean age is 60 years, most common liver abscess in developed world.
Amoebic: Most common type worldwide.
Hydatid: More common in sheep-rearing countries.

H: Fever, malaise, anorexia, night sweats, weight loss.
Right upper quadrant or epigastric pain, which may be referred to shoulder (diaphragmatic irritation).
Jaundice, diarrhoea, pyrexia of unknown origin.

E: Fever (continuous or spiking), jaundice.
Tender hepatomegaly (right lobe affected more commonly than left).
Dullness, ↓ breath sounds at right lung base (from reactive pleural effusion).

P: **Pyogenic:** Abscesses are typically polymicrobial, generated by an intense acute inflammatory response and are composed of neutrophils, macrophages, proteinaceous fluid, and bacterial debris.
Amoebic: Abscesses contain 'anchovy sauce' fluid of necrotic hepatocytes and trophozoites.
Hydatid cysts: Grow slowly, can hold litres of fluid, produce tissue damage by mechanical means and contain millions of infective stages, which are called hydatid sand (brood capsules and protoscolices).

I: **Bloods:** FBC (mild anaemia, leukocytosis, ↑ eosinophils in hydatid disease), LFT (↑ AlkPhos, ↑ bilirubin), ↑ ESR, ↑ CRP, blood cultures, amoebic and hydatid serology.
Stool microscopy, cultures: May pick up *E. histolytica* or tapeworm eggs.
Liver ultrasound or CT/MRI: Localises structure of mass.
CXR: Right pleural effusion or atelectasis, raised hemidiaphragm.

M: **Pyogenic:** Percutaneous (under ultrasound or CT guidance) aspiration (if small-sized) or catheter drainage (if moderate size) or occasionally surgical drainage (if large or multilocular abscesses). Broad-spectrum antibiotics (e.g. ceftriaxone and metronidazole) initially. Treatment of underlying cause.
Amoebic: Metronidazole and diloxanide furoate.
Hydatid: Surgical removal (pericystectomy) with mebendazole or albendazole treatment to reduce risk recurrence. In inoperable cases, drugs can be used.

C: Septic shock, rupture and dissemination (e.g. into biliary tract causing acute cholangitis, intrathoracic rupture or peritonitis), allergic sequelae or anaphylaxis from ruptured hydatid cyst.

P: Untreated pyogenic liver abscesses often fatal, complications have high mortality, amoebic abscesses have a better prognosis and usually have a quick response to therapy; hydatid cysts may recur after surgery (10%).

CONDITIONS

Liver resections

I: **Elective:** *Liver tumours*: Benign and malignant, primary and secondary. *Indications for colorectal metastases*: Solitary or metastases confined to localised area of the right lobe, with absent extrahepatic disease or limited to resectable local recurrence, and hepatic disease can be eradicated with a resection margin of > 5 mm, leaving at least three normal hepatic segments (or more if cirrhosis). *Infections*: Occasionally need resection (e.g. hydatid cysts). *Live-related liver donation*: Involving partial resection from donor and transplantation of the resected portion into the recipient.
Emergency: Trauma if techniques such as bimanual compression, suture ligation or packing have failed to control bleeding (i.e. resectional debridement of devitalised liver tissue).

A: The liver has four lobes, right, left, quadrate and caudate (the latter two anatomically part of the right lobe but functionally part of the left), and is divided into eight segments (of Couinaud), each with their branches of the arterial, venous and biliary systems. They are numbered I to VIII (from left to right). Resections can be segmental or nonsegmental. Normal livers have a great capacity to regenerate, with removal of up to 70% compatible with survival.
Vascular supply: The liver receives 1.5 L blood per minute from the hepatic artery (30%) and the portal vein (70%). Venous flow leads into the hepatic veins that drain into the vena cava.

I: Patients need to be selected through very strict eligibility criteria.
Imaging: CT, MRI, USS may be necessary for staging and planning resections.
Pre-op liver function score: For example, Childs–Pugh scoring (based on bilirubin, albumin, prothrombin time, presence of encephalopathy or ascites): cirrhosis precludes large resections due to the limited reserve of the residual cirrhotic liver.
Blood: FBC, U&Es, clotting, LFT.
Blood products: Blood and FFP should be crossmatched prior to operation as there is high risk of bleeding and transfusion requirement.

P: Usually carried out in specialist centres.
Incision: Rooftop incision below the ribcage running transversely across.
Cholecystectomy: Removal of gallbladder is often done prior to the resection.
Exploration: Intraoperative ultrasound is used to delineate the borders of a tumour and involvement of surrounding structures (e.g. biliary tree, vena cava).
Vascular occlusion: Temporary occlusion of inflow into the liver is achieved either by placing a tourniquet around the portal triad (Pringle's manoeuvre, up to 20 min) or selective vascular clamping of the Glisson's capsule of the segment.
Segmental resection: Dissection of the segment is commonly done with a harmonic scalpel/ultrasound dissector. Vessels and bile ducts are meticulously ligated. Finally, the resection surface should be carefully inspected for bile leakage or bleeding.
Closure of liver: Resection surfaces are sealed with either a collagen sponge or fibrin adhesive.
Closure: Three-layer closure with one continuous suture for all deep layers, one continuous suture for subcuticular fat, and staples, subcuticular or interrupted sutures for the skin.

C: Haemorrhage, biliary leakage, liver failure, sepsis (biliary or peritonitis), associated pulmonary complications (e.g. pleural effusion).

I: ~ 700 liver transplants are carried out annually in the UK. A highly specialised procedure, it is carried out in designated centres with multidisciplinary care including medical, surgical, anaesthetic and intensive care teams.

Elective: For end-stage liver disease (i.e. cirrhosis with Childs–Pugh class C). Liver disease with complications such as recurrent haemorrhage from varices, diuretic-resistant ascites, recurrent SBP, deteriorating synthetic function, hepatorenal syndrome or significantly reduced quality of life (e.g. PBC with intractable pruritus).

Metabolic diseases include Wilson's, α_1-antitrypsin deficiency and oxalosis.

In children, the most common indication is biliary atresia.

Emergency: Acute liver failure (most common causes are paracetamol overdose, viral hepatitis and idiosyncratic drug reactions). See criteria below.*

A: The liver is divided into eight segments, each with their branches of the arterial, venous and biliary systems. They are numbered I to VIII (from left to right).

Vascular supply: The liver receives blood from the hepatic artery and the portal vein. Venous flow leads into the hepatic veins, which drain into the vena cava.

I: **Pre-op:** Patients undergo a detailed and comprehensive work-up prior to be placed on the transplant waiting list. This includes a database of liver tests, liver biopsy, other blood tests, blood grouping, tissue typing, ABG, imaging (USS, CT of abdomen, head, chest), ECG and echocardiography, and other assessments, e.g. dental and psychiatry reviews. Once an organ has been allocated, the patient should be screened for sepsis (temperature, MSU, blood cultures, CXR and ascitic tap).

Post-op: Management is initially on ITU with close monitoring.

P: Liver transplantation involves the removal of the damaged liver and replacement with a graft in the native hepatic bed, i.e. orthoptic transplantation with anastomoses. In children, lack of donor organs has been addressed by performing splitting of donor organs (e.g. a left lateral segment of an adult donor organ can be transplanted into a child).

Donor organs: Most are from heart-beating donors that have suffered brainstem death. Objective measures of liver status or quality are lacking and, at present, subjective assessment by the surgeon of texture and fat content are used. Live related donors are increasingly being used, e.g. right hemihepatectomy of the donor. Donors and recipients are matched based on blood group and weight.

Organ retrieval: Occurs as part of multi-organ retrieval. The liver is mobilised and the hepatic artery, portal vein, bile duct and supra- and infrahepatic IVC dissected. Cannulae are inserted into the portal vein and aortic vessels are used to rapidly infuse the liver with cold preservative solution (University of Wisconsin solution prevents cell swelling). The liver is removed with its associated vessels and the biliary system flushed with University of Wisconsin solution. Maximum storage time is 15–18 h; with better results, the shorter the preservation period.

Recipient operation: Often technically demanding because of associated portal hypertension and coagulation abnormalities. Close invasive monitoring is required with transfusion of blood products, although this can be reduced by use of a cell saver (collects, washes and recycles RBCs).

Access: A *'mercedes-benz* incision' is used. The recipient's liver is mobilised and vasculature and bile duct dissected out.

Hepatectomy: Recipient hepatectomy involves clamping the IVC and in patients who are unlikely to tolerate the resulting fall in cardiac output, veno-venous bypass machines are used to divert flow from the IVC, returning via an axillary or jugular vein.

PROCEDURES

Graft anastomosis: The donor liver is then anastomosed via the suprahepatic IVC, infrahepatic IVC, portal vein, hepatic artery and then bile duct. The latter is formed by a direct end-to-end anastomosis or over a T-tube (removed after a few days). If the recipient bile duct is diseased, a Rouz-en-Y choledochoenterostomy may be performed.

Immunosuppression: Present regimens use either tacrolimus monotherapy or in combination with azathioprine and steroids. Monitoring for rejection is carried out by monitoring LFTs and biopsy of the transplanted liver (often via transjugular route).

C: Vascular: Haemorrhage. In 4–10%, hepatic artery thrombosis (a serious complication that usually necessitates retransplantation), more rarely portal vein thrombosis.

Biliary (in 12–19%)**:** Bile leakage, and later on anastomotic stenosis.

Infection: Opportunistic infections, e.g. fungal infections, CMV (10–20%).

Rejection:

Acute: Common and due to T-cells attacking the graft and treated by IV steroid boluses or antibody treatment (antithymocyte globulin).

Chronic (in < 5%): Occurs after the first year and is associated with progressive jaundice. Histology shows 'vanishing bile ducts' and small vessel occlusions, usually requires retransplantation.

Recurrent liver disease: Reinfection in the case of hepatitis B or C (if originally present) is common, the latter having the potential for an aggressive and rapidly progressive course. Hepatitis B can be managed with HB-Ig and immunisation. Other diseases that can recur include PBC, PSC and autoimmune hepatitis as well as recidivism in the case of alcoholic liver disease.

Complications of immunosuppression: Drug effects, infections, posttransplant malignancies, e.g. ↑ risk of skin cancers, lymphomas.

P: Survival rates are generally good with 85% at 1 year and 70% at 10 years.

*UK criteria for liver transplantation
Paracetamol overdose:
Arterial pH < 7.3 *or* PT > 100 s;
Grade III/IV encephalopathy; and
Creatinine > 300 μmol/L.
Non-paracetamol liver failure:
PT > 100 s *or* three of the following:
Age < 10 years or > 40 years;
Non-A, non-B hepatitis liver failure;
Drug- or halothane-induced liver failure;
Bilirubin > 300 μmol/L;
Jaundice to encephalopathy > 7 days;
PT > 50 s.

D: Primary malignant neoplasm of the lung. WHO classification of bronchocarcinoma: small cell (20%) and non-small cell (80%) – squamous cell carcinoma, adenocarcinoma, large cell carcinoma, adenosquamous carcinoma. Mesotheliomas are discussed in *Rapid Medicine*.

A: Factors such as smoking (active or passive) and asbestos exposure are thought to ultimately cause genetic alterations that result in neoplastic transformation.

A/R: Smoking, occupational exposures (polycyclic hydrocarbons, nickel, chromium, cadmium, radon), atmospheric pollution (urban > rural).

E: Most common fatal malignancy in the West (18% of cancer mortality worldwide), 35 000 deaths per year (UK), 3× more common in men (but ↑ in women).

H: May be asymptomatic with radiographic abnormality found (5%).
Due to primary: Cough, haemoptysis, chest pain, recurrent pneumonia.
Due to local invasion: For example, brachial plexus (Pancoast's tumour) causing pain in the shoulder or arm, left recurrent laryngeal nerve leading to hoarseness and bovine cough, oesophagus (dysphagia), heart: palpitations (arrhythmias).
Due to metastatic disease or paraneoplastic phenomena: Weight loss, fatigue, bone pain or fractures, fits.

E: There may be no signs.
Fixed monophonic wheeze.
Signs of lobar collapse or pleural effusion.
Signs of metastases (e.g. supraclavicular lymphadenopathy or hepatomegaly).

P: **Macro:** Tumours generally arise in main or lobar bronchi (see Fig. 22a), adenocarcinomas tend to occur more peripherally. Histological types as stated in **D**. The lung is also a site for secondary metastasis (see Fig. 22b).

I: **Diagnosis:** CXR, sputum cytology, bronchoscopy with brushings or biopsy, CT- or ultrasound-guided percutaneous biopsy, lymph node biopsy.
TNM staging: Based on tumour size, nodal involvement and metastatic spread, using CT chest, CT or MRI head and abdomen (or ultrasound), bone scan, PET scan. Invasive methods like mediastinoscopy or video-assisted thoracoscopy may be used.
Bloods: FBC, U&Es, Ca^{2+} (hypercalcaemia is common), AlkPhos (↑ bone metastases), LFT.
Pre-op: ABG, pulmonary function tests (FEV_1 > 80% predicted to tolerate a pneumonectomy, lung resection is contraindicated if FEV_1 < 30% predicted), V/Q scan, ECG, echocardiogram and general anaesthetic assessment.

M: Multidisciplinary discussion on tumour staging and optimal treatment modality. Important considerations (surgery is not appropriate for small cell cancer) are resectibility of the tumour (stages I and II disease, selectively IIIa) and operability (whether a patient is fit enough to undergo surgery). Frank discussion with the patient about the risks/benefits and the prognosis is vital. Only ~14% cases are considered for surgery.
Surgical:
Anaesthesia: A double-lumen endotracheal tube is used to isolate the lung to be operated on from the ventilatory circuit. Central line is placed ipsilateral to the lung to be operated on. Arterial line and urinary catheter are sited. Often, a thoracic epidural cathether is placed to give good regional analgesia.
Surgery: Rigid bronchoscopy is performed following induction of anaesthesia in the case of bronchial tumours. Antibiotic prophylaxis is used. The **thoracotomy** (usually posterolateral with the patient in a lateral decubitus position) is performed with gradual distraction of the ribs. The lung is mobilised and the

position of the tumour assessed and lymph nodes inspected. Branches of the bronchial tree, pulmonary artery and vein are identified and a **lobectomy** performed if appropriate (~60% of resections). **Bilobectomy** can be performed in the right lung, with preservation of the upper or lower lobe. **Sleeve resection** is used to avoid pneumonectomy (involves partial resection and reconstruction of bronchi). **Pneumonectomy** (25% of resections) involves removal of one lung. An anterior apical drain is placed to drain air, a posterior basal drain for blood or fluid.

Non-operable: Combined modality therapy with radiotherapy and chemotherapy improves survival. Small cell carcinomas are particularly suited for this treatment.

Palliation and terminal care: Includes laser therapy to bronchial tumours, endobronchial stents, management of complications and pain control.

C: Local invasion (e.g. brachial plexus, sympathetic chain, recurrent laryngeal nerve, SVC), metastases (commonly liver, bones and brain), pleural effusion, pulmonary haemorrhage, lobar or lung collapse, paraneoplastic syndromes (particularly common in small cell carcinomas, e.g. SIADH or ectopic ACTH production; squamous cell carcinomas are associated with hypercalcaemia of malignancy).

Of surgery: Lesion unresectable at surgery (should be < 5%).

Lobectomy: Air leaks are common, occasionally require re-operation.

Pneumonectomy: Considerable physiological strain due to whole of cardiac output passing through one lung, risks of cardiac arrhythmias, failure or MI, atelectasis and pneumonia, pulmonary oedema, bronchopleural fistula, bleeding, pulmonary embolus.

P: Depends on stage, but generally poor. Small cell carcinoma is often disseminated by the time of presentation. Overall 5-year survival < 5%. After resection for early stage disease ~25% 5-year survival. Mortality of lobectomy is < 2%, and mortality for pneumonectomy is 8%.

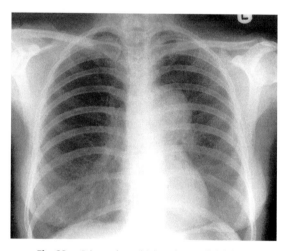

Fig. 22a   Primary bronchial carcinoma: left hilum.

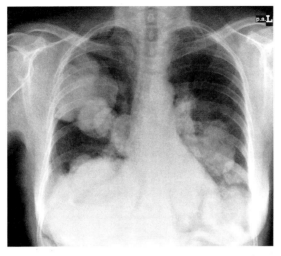

Fig. 22b   Secondary carcinoma of the lung: cannon ball metastasis.

Lymphoedema

D: Excessive accumulation of tissue fluid in the extracellular space due to impaired function of the lymphatic system.

A: **Primary:**
Milroy's disease: Autosomal dominant inherited condition (chromosome 5, vascular endothelial growth factor receptor-3 gene).
Distal obliteration: Also inherited, gene not yet known.
Proximal obstruction, hyperplasia and megalymphatics: Aetiology unknown.
Secondary: Following obstruction or destruction of lymphatic channels, e.g. infection with *Wuchereria bancrofti* (filariasis), TB, silica. Post radiotherapy or surgical excision of regional lymphatics in treatment of cancer, most commonly breast, also malignant infiltration of regional lymph nodes.

A/R: **Primary:** Milroy's disease is associated with other congenital abnormalities.

E: **Primary:** Uncommon, annual incidence 1/6000. 2–3× more common in females.
Secondary: Much more common. Worldwide, the most common cause is filariasis.

H: Can present at birth (Milroy's), during puberty (distal obliteration) or any age. Most often gradual swelling of one or both lower limbs, worse towards end of the day. In other cases swelling is of arm or genitalia. In megalymphatics, presentation can be with leaking skin vesicles, chylothorax or chylous ascites.

E: Early stages, skin oedema is pitting. Later, the skin becomes fibrotic, brawny and nonpitting, there may be weeping from vesicles. Ankles lose contour and toes become squared off. Thickened skin areas (condylomas) can develop.

P: Primary/congenital lymphoedema is an inherited deficiency of lymphatic vessels due to aplasia, hypoplasia (distal obliteration), hyperplasia or dilatation of the lymphatic channels usually affecting the lower limbs. In filariasis, the worm enters lymphatics and causes obstruction by inciting a fibrotic inflammatory reaction.

I: **Bloods:** FBC (for eosinophilia), U&Es, LFT, ESR.
Isotope lymphography: ^{99m}Tc-labelled colloid is injected SC into the first web space of the foot and the movement measured using a gamma counter.
Contrast lymphangiography: Now rarely performed.
CT or MRI scan: May highlight obstructive masses.
Tissue or lymph node biopsy.

M: **Conservative:** Skin or foot care, limb elevation, exercise, graduated compression stockings, massage, pneumatic massage devices are available. BP measurement or venesection should not be carried out from affected limbs.
Medical: Treatment of infection (e.g. antibiotics for cellulitis, antifungals for tinea pedis). Diuretics have no beneficial effects.
Surgical: Rarely used. Procedures used are debulking, bypass or ligation operations. Homan's operation involves creating skin flaps, excising SC tissue followed by resuturing of skin. Charles' reduction involves removal of skin and SC tissue, followed by skin grafting.

C: ↑ Fluid and protein renders skin prone to cellulitis, poor cosmesis, pain due to tissue swelling, reduced mobility, ulceration.

P: **Primary lymphoedema:** Good, usually responds to conservative measures.
Secondary lymphoedema: Depends on the aetiology.

I: Indications for mastectomy in breast cancer include:
A large (> 4 cm) or central subareolar breast tumour.
Multifocal tumours or widespread carcinoma in situ.
Patient choice.
Tumours fixed to underlying muscle or skin or those fungating through skin causing ulceration and bleeding ('toilet' mastectomy).

A: The mammary gland consists of 15–20 lobes radiating outwards from the nipple. Each lobe is separated from the other by fibrous septa and from the underlying muscle by the retromammary space. The base of the breast covers the 2nd to the 6th rib. The axillary tail runs upwards and laterally into the deep fascia at the lower border of pectoralis major muscle coming into close relation with the axillary vessels.
Vascular: The breast's arterial supply (and corresponding venous drainage) is from the perforating arteries of the internal thoracic, intercostal and axillary arteries.
Lymphatics: Lymphatics of the lateral half drains into the axillary nodes, comprising anterior, posterior, lateral, central and apical groups, while the medial half drain into the nodes along the internal thoracic artery. There is also some lymphatic drainage into the lymph vessels of the opposite breast.

I: **Pre-op:** Patients will have had diagnosis based on triple assessment of clinical examination, imaging (mammogram, ultrasound or if equivocal, MRI scan) and cytology/histological analysis by FNA or trucut biopsy. Ideally, a biopsy should confirm carcinoma prior to mastectomy. Staging investigations: CXR, bone scan, ultrasound abdomen $+/-$ CT scan. Neoadjuvant therapy, e.g. chemotherapy may be used prior to operation to downstage the tumour. FBC, U&Es, LFT, clotting, G&S or crossmatch. General anaesthetic assessment.
Post-op: DVT prophylaxis. Many patients require counselling or support.

P: Mastectomy involves removal of breast tissue, nipple/areola complex, an area of skin and axillary lymph nodes. In the past radical mastectomy (Halsted operation) involved removal of pectoralis major and minor; now a modified radical mastectomy is usually performed that preserves the pectoralis muscles with no difference in disease-free survival. Simultaneous axillary node sampling or clearance provides important staging information.
Access: An elliptical incision incorporating the primary tumour is made. The skin flaps are retracted exposing the superficial and deep fascia layers.
Modified radical mastectomy: Dissection of the clavi-pectoral fascia proceeds medially up to the costoclavicular ligament, allowing identification of the axillary vein. The entire breast is dissected free from the pectoralis major and rectus abdominis muscle aponeurosis using electrocautery and countertraction. The lateral border of the dissection is extended to lattisimus dorsi with careful preservation of the thoracodorsal and lateral thoracic nerves. The whole specimen is sent to histology including lymph nodes.
Axillary dissection: The loose areolar tissue of the axilla is dissected with careful identification and preservation of the axillary vessels, thoracodorsal nerve and artery to latissimus dorsi, and long thoracic nerve of Bell that supplies serratus anterior. Nodes removed include the lateral axillary (level I nodes) and the subscapular, with dissection continued medially to free the central nodal groups (level II nodes) and if necessary, the subclavicular nodes (level III nodes), by retraction or division of pectoralis minor, up to the costoclavicular ligament.
Closure: The wound is then thoroughly irrigated with saline, and two drains inserted via separate incisions, one catheter draining the axillary space and the second positioned superomedially to drain the surface area of pectoralis major muscle. The wound is closed with SC sutures and subcuticular sutures for the skin.

PROCEDURES

Reconstruction: Mastectomy can be combined with immediate reconstruction by latissimus dorsi or transverse rectus abdominus myocutaneous flap, with or without a subpectoral saline implant or expander. Alternatively, breast reconstruction can be delayed by several months.

C: Wound infection, serosanguinous collection, haemorrhage, nerve injury (e.g. long thoracic nerve, thoracodorsal nerve, intercostobrachial nerve).

Long-term: Poor cosmetic result, lymphoedema to ipsilateral arm, shoulder stiffness, psychological problems, tumour recurrence.

D: Small bowel diverticulum on the antimesenteric border of the ileum that is an embryological remnant. Follows the rule of twos: 'occurs in 2% of the population, ~ 2 feet from the ileocaecal junction, is 2 inches in length'.

A: In an embryo, the omphalomesenteric/vitelline duct connects the developing midgut to the yolk sac. Failure of the duct to completely regress during 5th–7th week can result in a persistent diverticulum or more rarely in an omphalomesenteric fistula, sinus, fibrous band or vitelline duct cyst.

A/R: None.

E: 2% of the population, males = females but twice as commonly symptomatic in males, at any age, but ~ 60% become so before the age of 10 years.

H: Most commonly asymptomatic.
PR bleeding (50%, most commonly in < 2-year-olds), usually painless dark or red blood (brick red) mixed with stool and can be major and associated with shock.
Abdominal pain due to diverticulitis/ulceration.
Symptoms of bowel obstruction (25%) due to volvulus or intussusception.
More rarely with mucoid or purulent discharge from the umbilicus.

E: Signs can be minimal. With bleeding there may be signs of shock. Pain due to inflammation/obstruction can vary depending on the position of the diverticulum, with guarding and rebound tenderness due to peritonism (can mimic acute appendicitis).

P: A true diverticulum (varies from 0.5 cm to 50 cm) as it is made up of all the layers of the bowel wall, lined by small intestinal mucosa but commonly contains heterotopic tissue (5% of asymptomatic and 60% of symptomatic cases), often gastric mucosa but duodenal, pancreatic or colonic mucosa can also be found. Ectopic gastric mucosa secretes acid that can cause erosion and result in bleeding.

I: **Bloods:** FBC, U&Es, clotting and G&S (if PR bleeding).
Isotope scan: ^{99m}Tc-pertechnetate is taken up by a Meckel's diverticulum if ectopic gastric mucosa is present (however, a negative scan does not exclude its presence). May be seen during barium contrast studies.
AXR, erect CXR: If signs of obstruction or perforation.
Mesenteric angiography: May be useful in cases of active bleeding; however, this may not be sensitive if bleeding is slow.

M: **Emergency** (bleeding or obstruction): Resuscitation with correction of fluid and electrolyte abnormalities.
Surgical: If bleeding or obstruction, surgical resection (diverticulectomy) with or without small bowel resection and division of bands.

C: Bleeding, obstruction secondary to an internal hernia around an omphalomesenteric band, inflammation (diverticulitis), intussusception or enterolith. Littre's hernia is one in which there is incarceration of a Meckel's diverticulum.

P: Usually good with appropriate management.

CONDITIONS

D: Malignancy arising from neoplastic transformation of melanocytes, the pigment forming cells of the skin. The leading cause of death from skin disease.

A: DNA damage in melanocytes caused by UV radiation results in neoplastic transformation. Inherited mutations identified in CDKN2A and CDK4 (tumour suppressor genes) in rare familial melanoma syndrome (autosomal dominant).

A/R: UV light exposure (sun exposure, especially history of blistering burning, use of tanning lamps, PUVA).
Fair skin, freckles, red/blond hair.
Family history (10%), giant congenital naevi.
Dysplastic naevus syndrome (multiple pigmented naevi, many > 5 mm, mainly on the trunk).
Congenital (e.g. xeroderma pigmentosum*).

E: Steadily increasing incidence, 6000 per year diagnosed in the UK, lifetime risk 1/80 in the USA. White races have a 20× risk to nonwhite races.

H: Change in size, shape or colour of a pigmented skin lesion, redness, bleeding, crusting, ulcerated.

E: **ABCDE criteria** for examining moles:
A Asymmetry
B Border irregularity/Bleeding
C Colour variation
D Diameter > 6 mm
E Elevation

P: 50% arise in pre-existing naevi, 50% in previously normal skin. Four histopathological types:
(1) **Superficial spreading (70%):** Typically arises in a pre-existing naevus, expands in radial fashion before vertical growth phase.
(2) **Nodular (15%):** Arises *de novo*, aggressive, no radial growth phase.
(3) **Lentigo maligna (10%):** More common in elderly with sun damage, large flat lesions, follows a more indolent growth course. Usually on the face.
(4) **Acral lentiginous (5%):** Arise on palms, soles and subungual areas. Most common type in nonwhite populations.

I: **Excisional biopsy:** For histological diagnosis and determination of Clark's levels or Breslow thickness.
Lymphoscintigraphy: Radioactive compound is injected around lesion and dynamic images are taken over the course of 30 min to trace the lymph drainage and the sentinel node(s).
Sentinel lymph node biopsy: Sentinel lymph nodes are dissected and histologically examined for metastatic involvement.
Staging: Imaging by USS, CT or MRI, CXR.
Bloods: LFT (liver is a common site of metastases).

M: **Primary prevention:** Limit sun overexposure, avoid sunburn, public education.
Surgical: Wide local excision, margin dependent on depth of invasion (< 1 mm: 1 cm, 1–4 mm: 2 cm margin). Skin grafting may be required.
Metastatic disease: Chemotherapy with dacarbazine (~ 20% respond). Immunotherapy (interferon α-2b, IL2).

C: Lymphoedema may result after block dissection of lymph nodes.

P: 5-year survival 90–95% for lesions < 1.4 mm depth, 40% with node-positive disease and mean survival of 9 months with metastatic disease.
Poorer prognostic indicators: ulceration, ↑ mitotic rate, trunk lesions compared to limb. Males poorer prognosis than females.

*Defect in DNA repair after UV light damage.

D: Malignancy of the nasopharynx.

A: There is a strong association with EBV with the incorporation of EBV antigens found in the tumour DNA.

A/R: Genetic susceptibility and environmental factors such as smoking, a high salt diet and alcohol are risk factors for disease development.

E: Rare, with a UK incidence of 2/100 000 though a higher incidence is seen in Oriental populations. Bimodal age of presentation 15–25 years and 40–60 years. 4× more common in men.

H: Nasal obstruction, 'nasal twang' to voice and epistaxis from local enlargement. Unilateral hearing loss and tinnitus develop if eustachian tube obstruction. Serous nasal discharge may indicate skull base invasion with diplopia, trismus and nasal regurgitation on cranial nerve involvement. Metastatic spread can present with bone pain, organ failure or paraneoplastic syndromes (uncommon).

E: Patients usually present late with palpable upper deep cervical nodes. Cranial nerve palsies may be demonstrable, most commonly cranial nerves V, VI, IX, X and XII.

P: **Macro:** Malignant growth originates from the lateral wall of the nasopharynx. **Micro:** 90% are squamous cell carcinoma or undifferentiated carcinoma with lymphoid tissue abundance within the stroma. **Spread:** Local spread can involve the eustachian tube, nose, skull base and cranial nerve invasion; lymphatics spread to deep cervical nodes. Blood-borne spread causes metastases to bone, lung, mediastinum and liver (rare).

I: **Indirect nasopharyngoscopy:** To assess the primary tumour. **Bloods:** FBC, U&Es, LFT, calcium, phosphate. **Lymph node or primary tumour biopsy:** For histological diagnosis. **CT/MRI scan:** Head and neck. **CXR:** Staging for metastatic spread to lungs. **Bone scintigraphy:** To detect for bone metastases. **EBV viral capsid antigen:** To confirm EBV exposure.

M: **Medical:** Initial chemotherapy with methotrexate, cisplatin, folinic acid and 5-fluorouracil is given prior to radiotherapy followed by adjuvant immuno-therapy with β-interferon. **Radiotherapy:** Radical radiotherapy is the treatment of choice targeting the primary tumour and the cervical lymph nodes. **Surgical:** Radical cervical node dissection can be performed if there are positive nodes on diagnosis or following a recurrence.

C: **From disease:** Nasal obstruction, eustachian tube obstruction, cranial nerve palsies, organ failure. **From radiotherapy:** Mucositis, hypothyroidism, secondary malignancy.

P: Much better in children than in adults (paediatric overall 5-year survival of 50–70% compared to an overall 5-year survival of 10–30% in adults).

CONDITIONS

D: Malignant tumour arising in the oesophagus. Two major histological types: squamous cell carcinoma and adenocarcinoma.

A: Aetiological risk factors are listed below.

A/R: **Squamous:** Alcohol, tobacco, Paterson–Kelly syndrome (also known as Plummer–Vinson syndrome), tylosis, achalasia, scleroderma, coeliac disease, certain nutritional deficiencies (vitamins A and C, trace elements) and dietary toxins (nitrosamines) also implicated.
Adenocarcinoma: GORD, Barrett's oesophagus (intestinal metaplasia of the distal oesophageal mucosa with a 1% incidence of adenocarcinoma per year).
E: Eighth most common malignancy (annual incidence in the UK is $\sim$7000–8000). 3$\times$ more common in males. Squamous cell carcinoma is more common in developing countries and shows considerable geographic variation (common in Northern China, Iran, parts of South Africa; whereas adenocarcinoma is more prevalent in the West (65% cases in the UK) and increasing at a rate of 5–10% per year (*Helicobacter pylori* eradication has been suggested as a possible contributing factor).

H: Often asymptomatic, causing symptoms only when locally advanced such as progressive dysphagia; initially worse for solids, regurgitation, cough or choking after food, voice hoarseness, pain (odynophagia), weight loss, fatigue (iron-deficiency anaemia).

E: No physical signs may be evident.
With metastatic disease there may be evidence of supraclavicular lymphaden-opathy, hepatomegaly, hoarseness due to recurrent laryngeal nerve involve-ment, signs of bronchopulmonary involvement.

P: **Macro:** Ulcerative, polypoid, fungating, or infiltrative tumours.
Micro: Squamous cell carcinomas appear as oval sheets of cells with keratinisa-tion and intercellular prickles (if differentiated). Adenocarcinoma usually de-velops in the lower oesophagus or gastro-oesophageal junction, may have an 'intestinal' (glandlike tubular growth pattern) or 'diffuse' (sheets and aggre-gates of tumour cells, with mucin and a compressed nucleus giving the cell a signet ring appearance) growth pattern. Spread is typically initially direct and longitudinal via submucosal lymphatics with early invasion of mediastinal struc-tures due to lack of an oesophageal serosa. Rare oesophageal tumours include lymphoma, melanoma and leiomyosarcoma.
Staging: TNM system.

I: **Endoscopy:** For brushings and biopsy, endoscopic ultrasound for tumour staging.
Imaging: Barium swallow, CXR.
Staging: CT chest and abdomen.
Other: Bronchoscopy (if risk of trancheo-bronchial invasion), lung function tests and ABGs, bone scan (if surgery is planned). Laparoscopy may be per-formed in cases of tumours involving the gastro-oesophageal junction.

M: Best managed at specialist centres with multidisciplinary expertise.
Surgical: $\sim$30% are suitable for surgical resection. Neoadjuvant chemora-diotherapy (e.g. cisplatin, 5-fluorouracil) may be beneficial in downstaging tumours prior to surgery. Operative approach depends on tumour location and extent of proposed lymphadenectomy. Examples are two- or three-stage subtotal oesophagectomy, or transhiatal total gastrectomy with Roux-en-Y jejunal reconstruction (the latter only for gastro-oesophageal junction tumours). Approaches by which these are carried out include the Sweet left thoraco-abdominal approach (low tumours), the Ivor–Lewis right thoracotomy and lapar-otomy (mid-lower third tumours) and transhiatal approaches, i.e. laparotomy and cervical approach (upper third tumours). Reconstruction is by mobilising

and pulling up the stomach on a vascular pedicle of the right gastroepiploic and right gastric arteries, isoperistaltic interposition of a section of the right colon, or Roux-en-Y jejunal reconstruction. Studies from Japan have shown improved survival with more extensive (three-field as opposed to two-field) lymphadenectomy.

Palliation: Luminal recannulisation by expandable stents or laser ablation techniques. Chemotherapy is associated with variable response rates, e.g. epirubicin, cisplatin and 5-fluorouracil.

Radiotherapy: Squamous cell carcinomas are more radiosensitive than adenocarcinomas.

C: Malnutrition, aspiration pneumonia, oesophageo-bronchial fistula.

Post-op: Pulmonary complications are the most common, e.g. atelectasis, pneumonia, others include anastomotic leakage (5–15%) – a serious complication that requires prompt and aggressive treatment, chylothorax, recurrent laryngeal nerve damage.

P: Overall poor with 5-year survival < 10%. After attempted curative resection 5-year survival is 20–25%. Unfortunately at present for most patients, medial survival is a matter of months.

Orthopaedic fixations

I: **External fixation:** Can refer to immobilisation of a fracture in a plaster, splint or on traction; however, more commonly refers to the fixation of bone fragments to an external device by the use of pins inserted into the fragments of a fracture. Indicated for open fractures if there is infection, or closed fractures if comminution precludes successful treatment by internal fixation or external cast.

Internal fixation: Failure to achieve adequate reduction or maintain reduction with external splintage methods, intra-articular fractures requiring good alignment, to provide early control of fractures where other measures would interfere with management of other injuries, to ensure rigid immobilisation and early mobilisation in certain fractures.

A: Bone is made up of an outer cortex and an inner medulla (containing the bone marrow). The substance of bone consists of bone matrix, osteoblasts and osteoclasts.

I: **Pre-op:** Patients have had radiographs of the affected bone indicating the need for fixation. FBC, U&Es and G&S are minimal pre-op blood investigations.
Post-op: Radiograph of affected bone to confirm reduction and fixation. Early mobilisation if appropriate.

P: A myriad of methods are available depending on the site and pattern of fracture.

External: Fixation is performed by placing threaded pins through the skin into the bony fragments, with external attachment to a rigid bar or frame – 'a fixator' – by clamps with multiaxial joints. These allow adjustment of position once the fixator has been applied.

Internal: Suitable only after open reduction of fractures. Methods include the use of **metal plates and screws:** there are two types of plates (neutralisation or dynamic) plates. The holes in the plates are offset so insertion of screws causes dynamic compression of underlying bone. Screws may be self-tapping or round-ended. **Intramedullary nails:** A hollow rod passed along the medullary cavity of a long bone fracture. Suitable for shaft fractures. Other methods include use of **transfixion screws, circumferential wires, Kirschner wires.**

C: Infection. Displacement of fixation. Soft tissue haematoma. Poor patient mobility resulting in muscle atrophy or DVT.

D: Degenerative condition of joint characterised by progressive loss of articular cartilage, pain and stiffness.

A: Can be classified according to distribution of joint sites involved.
Primary: Unknown. Likely to be multifactorial; 'wear-and-tear' concept proposed in the past.
Secondary: Other diseases can cause altered joint architecture and stability. Commonly associated diseases include:
(1) Developmental abnormalities (e.g. hip dysplasia, slipped femoral epiphysis).
(2) Trauma (e.g. previous fractures).
(3) Inflammatory (e.g. rheumatoid arthritis, gout, septic arthritis).
(4) Metabolic (e.g. alkaptonuria, haemochromatosis, acromegaly).

A/R: Age, previous joint injury, strenuous physical occupation.

E: Common, with 25% of >60 years symptomatic (70% have radiographic changes).

H: Joint pain or discomfort, stiffness after inactivity.
Difficulty with certain movements or feelings of instability.
Restriction to walking, climbing stairs and manual tasks.

E: Bone swelling at joint margins, e.g. Heberden's nodes (distal interphalangeal joints), Bouchard's nodes (at proximal interphalangeal joints).
Crepitus and pain during joint movement.
Restriction of range of joint movement.

P: Synovial joint cartilage fissuring and fibrillation. There is progressive loss of articular cartilage due to altered chondrocyte activity, subchondral sclerosis, bone cysts, osteophyte formation, patchy chronic synovial inflammation and fibrotic thickening of the joint capsules.

I: **Joint X-ray:** Radiographs of involved joints typically show four classic features:
(1) Joint space narrowing (due to cartilage loss);
(2) Subchondral cysts;
(3) Subchondral sclerosis; and
(4) Osteophytes.
Severity of radiological changes is not a good indicator of symptom severity.
Synovial fluid analysis: Not indicated in most cases. Clear synovial fluid, viscous with low cell count and possibly cartilage fragments.

M: Treatment goals include symptom relief, optimising joint function, minimising disease progression and limiting disability.
Medical: Analgesia with paracetamol, codeine, NSAIDs, COX-2 inhibitors or quinine. Topical capsaicin may provide some benefit. Intra-articular injection of steroids and hyaluronic acid provides good but transient symptomatic relief.
Supportive: Patient education. Encourage lifestyle changes (e.g. weight loss, exercise). Physiotherapy, occupational therapy, and psychosocial support.
Surgical: Various techniques can provide benefits like arthroscopic irrigation, osteophyte removal, joint replacement and joint fusion.
Rehabilitation: Requires concerted effort from clinicians, physiotherapists, occupational therapists and patient to encourage return to normal physical activity.

C: Pain, disability, nerve entrapment syndromes and falls from reduced mobility.

P: Although symptoms may improve or worsen in phases, disease evolution is usually slow, with the natural history depending on the joint site involved.

CONDITIONS

Osteomyelitis

CONDITIONS

D: Infection of the bone leading to inflammation, necrosis and new bone formation. Can be acute, subacute or chronic.

A: Bacterial infection from direct inoculation from skin, e.g. trauma, operative or chronic skin ulcers, haematogenous spread or from associated septic arthritis.

A/R: Diabetes, immunosupression, IV drug use, prostheses and sickle-cell anaemia.

E: Most common in young children, < 20% cases in adults. Incidence of 2 : 10 000.

H: Pain in the affected area. Associated fever, malaise or rigors. There may be a history of a preceding skin lesion, sore throat, trauma or operation. There may be no localising signs in infants, presenting with fever, drowsiness and irritability.

E: Localised erythema, tenderness, swelling and warmth. Movement of the affected limb is limited by pain. Seropurulent discharge from an associated wound or ulcer.

P: Most common causative organism in children is *Staphylococcus aureus* and Group A *Streptococcus*; *S. aureus* in adults; coliforms can cause osteomyelitis in neonates. The disease can affect any bone.
Acute haematogenous: Bone seeded from sepsis or bacteraemia often settles in the metaphyseal region, possibly because the vessels here act as end arterioles, trapping the organisms. Acute inflammation develops causing pain due to ↑ intraosseous pressure, initially in the medulla. Pus then passes through the cortex to form a subperiosteal abscess, causing stripping of the periosteum from the underlying bone and stimulating new bone formation. This new bone (or 'involucrum') can surround a necrotic area that consists of sequestra of dead bone in pus and granulation tissue.
Chronic: Often associated with overlying chronic skin infection. An imprisoned sequestrum can cause a chronic seropurulent discharge. May be dormant with recurrent flares of redness, pain and swelling. Cierny–Mader classification is: type I: medullary; type II: superficial; type III: localised; type IV: diffuse.

I: **Bloods:** FBC, blood culture, ESR, CRP.
Swabs of wound or discharge: To identify the causative organism.
Radiographs: Will show no abnormality in the first 10 days, after which there is metaphyseal mottling, periosteal bone formation, sequestra or abscesses (see Fig. 23).
Radioisotope bone scan: Identifies areas of raised activity prior to X-ray changes.

M: **Medical:** Early IV antibiotic treatment may be successful. Initial empiric therapy is modified according to microbial culture results, e.g. flucloxacillin and fusidic acid, with cephalosporins for gram-negative cover in children. Antibiotic treatment may be needed for several weeks. Adequate analgesia and splinting is used to control pain. Any wounds are dressed regularly.
Surgical: Drainage of accessible abscesses, debridement of necrotic tissue and removal of associated implants (bacterial biofilms make it extremely difficult to ever sterilise the prosthesis). External fixation may be necessary for skeletal stabilisation with plastic surgery to restore soft tissue cover.

C: Septicaemia, spread to joint, recurrence, pathological fracture, growth disturbance in children, skin sinuses over sites of bone infection.

P: With appropriate treatment, prognosis is excellent for acute osteomyelitis, chronic cases can be more problematic with late recurrent osteomyelitis seen in 5% patients.

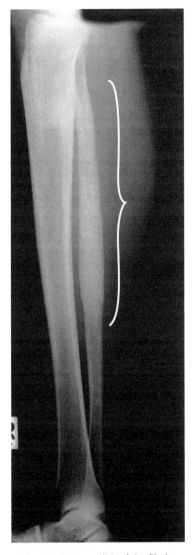

Fig. 23   Osteomyelitis of the fibula.

D: Most common primary bone tumour, arising from mesenchymal cells.

A: 90% idiopathic, 10% secondary to underlying bone disorder.

A/R: In the elderly, osteosarcoma is commonly associated with Paget's disease. Associated with rare syndromes of oncogene mutation such as germ-line retinoblastoma and Li–Fraumeni syndrome.

E: Rare, incidence 3/million, 75% cases 10–25 years, smaller peak in the elderly, more common in males.

H: Painful limb with associated swelling, most commonly femur in young patients, may wake the patient at night.
Pathological fracture is a common first presentation.

E: Painful swelling in the region of the metaphysis of a long bone or in association with flat bones in Paget's disease.
Reduced range of motion if there is joint involvement.
May have chest signs as 20% have pulmonary metastases on presentation.

P: Osteosarcomas most commonly arise in the medullary cavity of the metaphyseal ends of long bones. Can develop into big bulky tumours frequently destroying overlying cortex, producing a soft tissue mass. Stromal cells lay down osteoids, which may be visible histologically or using an electron microscope.

I: **Bloods:** AlkPhos (↑), Ca^{2+}, PO_4^{2-} LDH (↑ indicates poor prognosis), protein electrophoresis (to exclude myeloma), FBC, LFT.
Radiography: Large destructive mass with diffuse margins, may be lytic or sclerotic, rays of ossification within the tumour causing a 'sunburst' effect. The periosteum may be lifted inducing it to lay down bone and producing the classic triangular shadow of the 'Codman triangle'.
Biopsy: Usually via an open incision or trephine. Frozen sections should be taken to ensure accurate sampling.
MRI scan: Allows clear imaging of the margins of the tumour and the extent of intramedullary involvement. Necessary for the planning of curative surgery.
Staging: Bone scan, CXR.

M: **Chemotherapy:** Biggest advance in improving prognosis. Used as neoadjuvant or adjuvant therapy to shrink the tumour and prevent recurrence. Doxorubicin, cisplatin and high-dose methotrexate are commonly used agents. Granulocyte colony-stimulating factor may be needed to prevent neutropenia.
Surgical: Definitive curative resection requires good clear margins. There is a wide variety of limb salvage procedures including prosthesis and bone grafts. Amputation may be indicated in large tumours if limb salvage is impossible.

C: Pathological fractures, metastases.

P: Much improved. 5-year survival is 60–70%. Multifocal osteosarcomas or those in association with Paget's disease have a poorer outcome.

D: Malignancy arising from the exocrine or endocrine tissues of the pancreas.

A: Unknown. 5–10% are hereditary in nature (MEN, HNPCC, FAP, Gardner, von Hippel–Lindau syndromes are associated).

A/R: Increasing age, smoking, DM, chronic pancreatitis, dietary factors (low in fresh fruits and vegetables).

E: Increasing in incidence (8–12/100 000). 2× more males, peak age 60–80 years.

H: Clinical diagnosis of pancreatic cancer is often difficult as the initial symptoms are often quite nonspecific. These include anorexia, malaise, nausea, epigastric pain. Later, weight loss, DM, jaundice.

E: Signs of weight loss, epigastric tenderness or mass.
Jaundice and a palpable gallbladder (Courvoisier's law: a palpable gallbladder with painless jaundice is unlikely to be caused by gallstones).
In patients with metastatic spread, there may be hepatomegaly. Trousseau's sign is an associated superficial thrombophlebitis.

P: **Macro:** ~75% occur within the head or neck of the pancreas (where it can present as a periampullary tumour), 15–20% occur in the body and 5–10% occur in the tail. Spread is local and to the liver.
Micro: 80% are adenocarcinomas of the ductal epithelium, other types include adenosquamous, mucinous cystadenocarcinomas. Endocrine tumours include insulinomas, glucagonomas and gastrinomas.

I: **Bloods:** Tumour markers CA19-9 and CEA can be elevated (former more specific, but neither are diagnostic). If causing obstructive jaundice, ↑ bilirubin, ↑ AlkPhos, clotting may be deranged.
Imaging: Ultrasound, CT +/− guided biopsy, MRI and MRCP are all useful in staging the disease. ERCP may allow biopsy/bile cytology +/− stenting.
Other: Staging laparoscopy or intraoperative ultrasound.

M: **Medical:** Most patients with disease who are not amenable to curative resection undergo palliative management. This may involve radiotherapy or chemotherapy with 5-fluorouracil, gemcitabine. Pain relief can be carried out by medical analgesia, or coeliac plexus block. For obstructive jaundice, endoscopic stent insertion or a choledochojejunostomy is carried out. For duodenal obstruction an endoscopic stenting or a gastrojejunostomy is carried out.
Surgery: Tumours on the body and tail are often unresectable at presentation. *Pancreaticoduodenectomy (Whipple procedure):* For tumours of the head (< 3 cm and no nodal metastases). Involves en bloc resection of the pancreatic head, 1st–3rd parts of the duodenum; the distal antrum; and the distal common bile duct. The GI tract is reconstructed with a gastrojejunostomy. The common bile duct and residual pancreas are anastomosed into a segment of small bowel.
Pylorus-preserving pancreaticoduodenectomy: Alternative procedure. Sparing the pylorus allows for more physiological emptying of the stomach.

C: Unresectable disease, pain, obstructive jaundice, pruritus, cholangitis, diabetes, splenic vein thrombosis, malignant ascites.
From surgery: Anastomotic leaks, pancreatic fistulas, brittle diabetes.

P: Fewer than 5% of all patients are still alive 5 years later. The median survival of all patients after initial diagnosis is 4–6 months. In patients able to undergo a successful curative resection the median survival ranges from 12 to 19 months, and the 5-year survival rate is 15–20%. Patients with periampullary and endocrine tumours have a better prognosis.

CONDITIONS

Pancreatitis, Acute

CONDITIONS

D: Acute inflammation of the pancreas.

A: **Most common:** Gallstones, alcohol (80% cases).
Others: Drugs (e.g. steroids, azathioprine, thiazides, valproate), trauma, ERCP or abdominal surgery, infective (e.g. mumps, EBV, CMV, Coxsackie B, mycoplasma), hyperlipidaemia, hyperparathyroidism, anatomical (e.g. pancreas divisum, annular pancreas), idiopathic.

A/R: As above.

E: Common. Annual UK incidence $\sim 10/10\,000$. Peak age is 60 years; in males alcohol-induced is more common while in females, principal cause is gallstones.

H: Severe epigastric or abdominal pain (radiating to back, relieved by sitting forward, aggravated by movement).
Associated with anorexia, nausea and vomiting.
There may be a history of gallstones or alcohol intake.

E: Epigastric tenderness, fever.
Shock, tachycardia, tachypnoea.
Jaundice may be present.
↓ Bowel sounds (due to ileus).
If severely haemorrhagic, Turner's sign (flank bruising) or Cullen's sign (periumbilical bruising).

P: Insult results in activation of proenzymes within the duct/acini resulting in tissue damage and inflammation. Varies in severity from mild glandular and interstitial oedema to frank parenchymal necrosis and haemorrhage with release of inflammatory mediators into the systemic circulation. Saponification (foaming) may be seen due to action of lipases and proteases on pancreatic tissue.

I: **Bloods:** ↑ Amylase (usually $> 3\times$ normal), ↑ serum lipase, FBC (↑ WCC, ↑ haematocrit), U&Es, ↑ glucose, ↑ CRP > 100 at 48 h is prognostically severe, ↓ Ca^{2+}, LFT (deranged if due to gallstone pancreatitis or alcohol), ABG (for hypoxia or metabolic acidosis). See modified Glasgow criteria below.
USS: For gallstones or biliary dilatation. Pancreas often difficult to visualise due to overlying bowel gas.
Erect CXR: Mainly to exclude other causes of an acute abdomen. There may be pleural effusion.
AXR: To exclude other causes of acute abdomen. Psoas shadow may be lost. CT scanning for severe cases.
Assessment of severity: Modified Glasgow[*] or Ranson's criteria[†] (for alcohol induced pancreatitis), CRP.
Note: Amylase level does not correlate with severity.

M: **Intensive supportive care:** Fluid and electrolyte resuscitation and close monitoring. Nil by mouth. Urinary catheter and NG tube. Analgesia. Later, nutritional support may be necessary. Prophylactic antibiotics have not been shown to reduce mortality but are often given. If it is gallstone pancreatitis, stone removal by ERCP can be considered in severe cases or with cholestatic jaundice.
Early detection and treatment of complications: Monitor respiratory function, renal function and clotting. Management in ITU may be necessary for severe cases.
Surgical: For necrotising pancreatitis. Drainage and debridement of all necrotic tissues should be performed.

C: **Local:** Pancreatic necrosis, pseudocyst, abscess, pancreatic ascites. In the long term, chronic pancreatitis (with diabetes and malabsorption).

Systemic: Multiorgan dysfunction, sepsis, renal failure, ARDS.

 20% follow severe fulminating course with high mortality (pancreatic necrosis associated with 70% mortality), 80% run milder course (but still 5% mortality).

*Modified Glasgow criteria:
WCC $>15 \times 10^9$/L, glucose >10 mmol/L, urea >16 mmol/L, AST >200 unit/L, $pO_2 < 8$ kPa, albumin >32 g/L, $Ca^{2+} < 2$ mmol/L, LDH >600.

†Ranson's criteria:
On admission: WCC $>16 \times 10^9$/L, age >55, AST >250, LDH >350, glucose >11 mmol/L.
During first 48 h: $pO_2 < 8$kPa, $Ca^{2+} < 2$mmol/L, urea >16 mmol/L, base deficit >4, haematocrit fall $>10\%$, fluid sequestration >600 ml.

CONDITIONS

CONDITIONS

D: Chronic inflammation of the pancreas with permanent structural changes leading to impaired endocrine and exocrine function and recurrent abdominal pain.

A: **Major:** Alcohol.
Others: Idiopathic in 20%. Rare: exogenous toxins, cystic fibrosis, haemachromatosis, α_1-antitrypsin deficiency, pancreatic duct obstruction (acute pancreatitis, pancreas divisum, pancreatic duct anomalies), hyperparathryroidism.

A/R: As above.

E: Annual UK incidence is about 1/100 000; prevalence is about 3/100 000. Mean age 40–50 years in alcohol-associated disease.

H: Recurrent severe epigastric pain, radiating to back, relieved by sitting forward. Exacerbated by eating or after an episode of binge drinking.
May be associated with bloating and pale offensive stools (steatorrhoea).
Diarrhoea, weight loss, thirst and polyuria.

E: Epigastric tenderness.
There may be epigastric fullness (due to pseudocyst).
Signs of weight loss, malnutrition and alcohol abuse.

P: Disruption of normal glandular architecture due to chronic inflammation and fibrosis, calcification, ductal dilatation, cyst and stone formation.

I: **Bloods:** Glucose (↑ may indicate endocrine dysfunction), glucose tolerance test. Amylase and lipase (usually normal), LFT (↑ if common bile duct obstruction).
USS: Percutaneous or endoscopic.
ERCP or MRCP: Early changes include main duct dilatation and stumping of branches. Late manifestations are duct strictures with alternating dilatation ('chain of lakes' appearance).
AXR: Pancreatic calcification may be visible (see Fig. 24).
CT scan: Pancreatic cysts, calcification.
Tests of pancreatic exocrine function: Faecal elastase.

M: **General:** Dietary advice and alcohol abstinence.
Acute: Analgesics for exacerbations of pain.
Chronic: Pain management may need specialist pain clinic, treatment of diabetes (e.g. insulin). Pancreatic enzyme replacements (e.g. Creon, Pancrease). Endoscopic stenting of strictures may be possible.
Pain control: As the majority of sensory nerves to the pancreas transverse the coeliac ganglia and splanchnic nerves, both coeliac plexus block and transthoracic splanchnicectomy offer variable degrees of pain relief.
Surgical: Indicated if medical management has failed. Options include proximal resection (pancreaticoduodenectomy) or lateral pancreaticojejunal drainage (Puestow procedure).

C: **Local:** Pseudocysts, biliary duct stricture, duodenal obstruction, pancreatic ascites, pancreatic carcinoma.
Systemic: DM, steatorrhoea, hyperglycaemic coma. Many develop chronic pain syndromes and become dependent on strong analgesics.

P: Surgery improves symptoms in 60–70% but results are often not sustained. Life expectancy is reduced by 10–20 years.

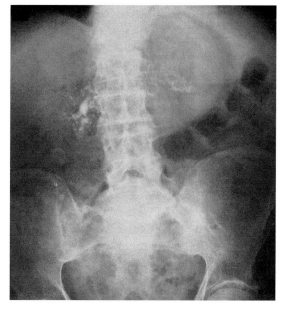

Fig. 24   Chronic pancreatitis with calcification within the pancreas.

CONDITIONS

Paralytic ileus

CONDITIONS

D: Functional bowel obstruction due to atony and disruption of normal peristalsis.

A: **Post-op ileus following intra-abdominal surgery.**
Metabolic: Hypokalaemia, hypomagnesaemia, ketoacidosis, uraemia, porphyria, heavy metal poisoning.
Inflammation: Response to a local inflammatory process, e.g. appendicitis.
Diffuse peritonitis: Bacterial or chemical.
Retroperitoneal pathology: Haematoma, pancreatitis.
Drugs: Opioids, antipyschotics, anticholinergics, Parkinson's disease medications.
Neuropathic disorders: Diabetes, multiple sclerosis, scleroderma.
Ogilvie's syndrome: Colonic pseudo-obstruction, associated with long-term debility, chronic disease, immobility and polypharmacy.

A/R: See above.

E: Depending on aetiology but a common problem in surgical patients.

H: Failure to open bowels, constipation. Initally, abdominal distension without pain, but later symptoms may mimic those of true obstruction.
History relevant to cause, e.g. recent surgery.

E: Abdominal distension. Bowel sounds may be reduced or absent. Mild tenderness, if guarding or rebound tenderness, peritonitis should be diagnosed. There may be faecal impaction on rectal examination.

P: Post-op paralytic ileus is related to several factors: sympathetic overactivity, the effects of handling bowel, changes in mucosal permeability, potassium depletion and peritoneal irritation by blood. Reflex paralytic ileus is thought to be due to interference with the autonomic nervous supply while peritonitis results in the toxin release and paralysis of the intrinsic nerve plexuses. Paralytic ileus may result in fluid, electrolyte and protein loss in the bowel lumen; combined with gaseous dilatation, can result in subsequent impairment of mesenteric blood supply and toxin absorption.

I: As appropriate to patient's status and aetiology. May include:
Blood: FBC, U&Es, Mg^{2+}, ESR and CRP.
Imaging: Erect CXR and AXR, CT scan: May show distension of bowel, faecal impaction. Caecal diameter > 12 cm significantly ↑ risk of perforation. A water-soluble contrast enema may help exclude a mechanical obstruction.

M: As appropriate, depending on aetiology, approaches used include:
Conservative: Nil by mouth, NG tube if vomiting, IV fluid replacement and correction of electrolyte imbalances. If faecal impaction, may respond to enema, manual evacuation or placement of a flatus tube for decompression.
Medical: Treatment of the underlying cause (e.g. infection). In the absence of mechanical obstruction, persistent paralytic ileus may respond to prokinetic agents such as metoclopramide, domperidone or erythromycin.
Surgical: If the bowel is severely distended and there is danger of perforation, decompression and stoma formation may be needed.

C: Bowel perforation, most commonly caecal (40% mortality), peritonitis.

P: Usually responds to conservative measures. Colonic psuedo-obstruction can be a chronic problem in older patients.

D: Penile malignancy, most commonly squamous cell carcinoma of the penile skin.

A: Chronic irritation is main risk factor. Human papilloma virus also implicated.

A/R: Condyloma acuminata (e.g. warts, human papilloma virus), chronic infection of the foreskin (balanitis), smoking. Balanitis xerotica obliterans (a form of lichen sclerosus, a chronic inflammatory condition of the glans or foreskin), erythroplasia of Queyrat (a form of carcinoma in situ of the glans skin), Bowen's disease (intraepithelial carcinoma of the penile shaft).

E: Rare, most commonly seen in elderly men (50–70 years), < 0.5% of adult male cancers.

H: The patient may report a slowly enlarging lesion, often painless leading to delay in seeking medical attention, there may be associated bleeding or discharge.

E: Most often occurs on the glans penis or inner surface of the foreskin, early as a painless red lesion, later as an exophytic papilliferous or nodular growth or ulcer, often with secondary infection causing a discharge or offensive smell. Inguinal lymphadenopathy is present in up to 50% but often due to the associated infection or inflammation with only 30–60% of these having evidence of tumour spread.

P: These are squamous cell carcinomas, with three histological grades G1, G2 and G3.
Stage I: Localised to the glans or foreskin.
Stage II: Involvement of the corpora.
Stage III: Spread to inguinal nodes.
Stage IV: Distant metastases.
A variant is giant condyloma of Buschke–Löwenstein that spreads locally with a characteristic sharply defined deep margin.

I: **Biopsy:** Punch or excisional biopsy to establish diagnosis (differential: condylomata acuminata, syphilitic chancre or rarely chancroid).
Imaging: CT or MRI scanning for evidence of spread.

M: **Prevention:** Circumcision at a young age, good hygiene, appropriate treatment of erythroplasia of Queyrat (5-fluorouracil cream or local laser photocoagulation).
Surgical: For stage I and II, partial amputation with 2 cm proximal disease-free margins. In more advanced cases, total penectomy with formation of a perineal urethrostomy.
Inguinal nodes: Palpable nodes should be treated with antibiotics after treatment of the initial lesion as they may be a reactive response to infection. If persistent, bilateral ilioinguinal block dissection is performed, and if involved, this may still be curative. Prophylactic dissection of impalpable nodes has not been associated with ↑ survival although superficial node dissection is used for staging.
Radiotherapy: Local radiotherapy may be used for early stage disease if the tumour is not large, invasive or involving the urethra, or as part of combined modality therapy for palliation of advanced stage disease.
Chemotherapy: Usually restricted to cases of systemic spread, agents such as cisplatin and bleomycin are used, although often with only partial responses.

C: Psychological morbidity of penectomy.
From inguinal node dissection: Lymphoedema, wound breakdown.

P: 5-year survival rate is 80% (stage I), 50% (nodal involvement) and 0% (metastases).

CONDITIONS

CONDITIONS

D: Ulceration of areas of the GI tract caused by exposure to gastric acid and pepsin. Most commonly gastric and duodenal (can also occur in oesophagus and Meckel's diverticulum).

A: Cause is an imbalance between damaging action of acid and pepsin and mucosal protective mechanisms.
Common: Very strong association with *Helicobacter pylori* (present in 95% of duodenal and 70–80% of gastric ulcers), NSAID use.
Rare: Zollinger–Ellison syndrome.

A/R: Weak association with smoking, alcohol, genetic susceptibility, blood group O.

E: Common. Annual incidence is about 1–4/1000. More common in males. Duodenal ulcers have a mean age in the thirties, while gastric ulcers have a mean age in the fifties. *H. pylori* is usually acquired in childhood and the prevalence is roughly equivalent to age in years.

H: **Epigastric abdominal pain:** Relieved by antacids.
Symptoms have a variable relationship to food (e.g. if worse soon after eating, more likely to be gastric ulcers; if worse several hours later, more likely to be duodenal).
May present with complications (e.g. haematemesis, melaena).

E: May be no physical findings.
Epigastric tenderness.
Signs of complications (e.g. anaemia, succession splash in pyloric stenosis).

P: **Pathogenesis:** There is a strong correlation with *H. pylori* infection, but it is unclear how the organism causes formation of ulcers.
Macro: Ulceration (usually < 3 cm) with well-defined edges and a grey-white floor. There may be surrounding erythema or a visible bleeding vessel.
Micro: Four layers (Askanazy's zones):
Layer 1: Thin exudate of fibrin and inflammatory cells
Layer 2: Necrotic tissue layer
Layer 3: Inflammatory granulation tissue
Layer 4: Dense fibrous tissue

I: **Bloods:** FBC (for anaemia), amylase (to exclude pancreatitis), U&Es, clotting screen (if GI bleeding), LFT, crossmatch if actively bleeding.
Endoscopy: Four quadrant gastric ulcer biopsies to rule out malignancy; duodenal ulcers need not be biopsied.
Rockall scoring for severity after a GI bleed based on age, systolic BP, heart rate, comorbidity, underlying diagnosis and stigmata of recent haemorrhage.
Testing for H. pylori:
^{13}C-Urea breath test: Radio-labelled urea given by mouth and detection of ^{13}C in the expired air. For confirming eradication after treatment.
Serology: IgG antibody against *H. pylori*, confirms exposure but not eradication, as IgG may remain positive.
Camylobacter-like organism test: Gastric biopsy is placed with a substrate of urea and a pH indicator, if *H. pylori* is present, ammonia is produced from the urea and there is a colour change (yellow to red).
Histology of biopsies: Difficult to visualise *H. pylori*.

M: **Acute:** Resuscitation if perforated or bleeding, and proceeding endoscopic or surgical treatment.
Endoscopy: Haemostasis by injection sclerotherapy, laser or electrocoagulation.
Surgical: If perforated, ulcer can be oversewn or an omental patch can be placed over it. Haemorrhage is controlled by suturing the affected vessels (usually gastroduodenal artery). In chronic cases where ulcer-related bleeding

cannot be controlled, partial gastrectomy and/or vagotomy and sometimes trans-arterial embolisation can be attempted.

Medical: *H. pylori* eradication with 'triple therapy' for 1–2 weeks: Various combinations are recommended made up of one PPI/ranitidine bismuth sulphate and two antibiotics (e.g. clarithromycin + amoxicillin, metronidazole + tetracycline).

If not associated with *H. pylori*: Treat with PPIs or H_2-antagonists. Stop NSAID use (especially diclofenac), use misoprostol (prostaglandin E_1 analogue), if NSAID use is necessary.

C: **Major complication rate:** 1% per year including haemorrhage (haematemesis, melaena, iron-deficiency anaemia), perforation, obstruction/pyloric stenosis (due to scarring, penetration, pancreatitis).

P: Overall lifetime risk ~10%. Generally good as peptic ulcers associated with *H. pylori* can be cured by eradication.

Perineal abscesses and fistulae

CONDITIONS

D: **Perineal abscess:** A pus collection in the perineal region.
Perineal fistula: An abnormal chronically infected tract communicating between the perineal skin and either the anal canal or rectum.

A: Bacteria, often tracking from anal glands cause infection that the body's defenses do not overcome, with fistulae developing as a complication of abscess. The latter are also a complication of Crohn's disease, where multiple perineal fistulae may develop (pepperpot perineum).

R: May be associated with IBD, DM or malignancy (rectal carcinoma).

E: Common.

H: Constant throbbing pain in the perineum and intermittent discharge (mucus or faecal staining) near the anal region.
Enquire about personal and family history of IBD.

E: Localised tender perineal mass (may be fluctuant) or a small skin lesion near the anus corresponding to the opening of a fistula.
PR examination: An area of induration corresponding to the abscess or fistula tract may be felt. Not always possible due to pain or sphincter spasm. Examination under sedation or general anaesthesia may be warranted.
Goodsall's rule: Rule of thumb to correlate location of internal fistula opening based on location of external fistula opening. If external opening is anterior to the anal canal (i.e. lies anterior to a transverse anal line), the fistula runs radially and directly into the anal canal. The exception to this is a fistula 3 cm away. This and any other fistula whose external opening is posterior to the anal canal (i.e. lies posterior to a transverse anal line) will follow a curved path, opening internally in the posterior midline (see Fig. 25a).

P: **Abscess types:** Classified according to location: submucous, SC, intersphincteric, ischiorectal and pelvirectal abscesses.
Fistula types: Park's classification as superficial, intersphincteric, transsphincteric, suprasphincteric or extrasphincteric, or alternatively as low anal (below puborectalis) or high anal (at or above puborectalis) and pelvirectal (involving levator ani). (See Fig. 25b.)

I: **Blood:** FBC, CRP, ESR, blood culture.
Imaging: MRI is extremely useful in allowing detailed study of the often complex and deep pus-filled tracts. Allows for surgical planning ensuring complete excision.
Endoanal USG: Also used, though less useful than MRI.

M: Requires surgical treatment under general anaesthesia. Analgesia.
Open drainage of abscess: Most common procedure is deroofing of abscess. A cross-shaped 'cruciate' incision is made over the abscess to open it. The loculi of pus are digitally broken up and all necrotic material is extracted. Packs soaked in antiseptic, e.g. Kaltostat are then inserted into the cavity.
Laying open of fistula: A probe is used to gently explore the tract. Hydrogen peroxide or methylene blue can be injected into the external opening to demonstrate the internal opening.
Low fistulae: Treatment with a fistulotomy involves cutting down on and laying open the tract, curetting away granulation tissue and allowing healing by secondary intention. Extreme care must be taken to avoid damage to the sphincter muscles.
High fistulae: For fistulae involving the upper half of the sphincter complex, where muscle division would cause incontinence, a seton is used. This is a nonabsorbable suture that is threaded through the fistula tract. It first allows drainage of sepsis. It can then be tightened, whereby it slowly cuts through the sphincter in a manner that preserves continence. An alternative procedure

is the excision of the external part of the fistula and closure of the internal opening by a mucosal advancement flap.

Antibiotics: Samples need to be taken from the abscess to be cultured. A common initial regimen is cefuroxime and metronidazole.

C: Recurrence. Damage to the internal anal sphincter and incontinence. Persisting pain.

P: High recurrence rate without complete excision.

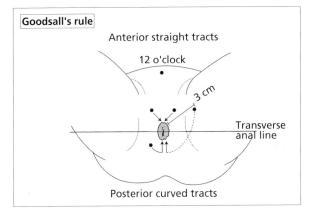

Fig. 25a

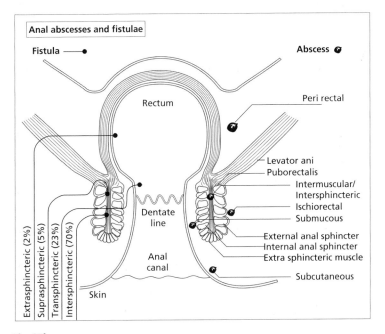

Fig. 25b

CONDITIONS

D: Peritonitis is inflammation of the peritoneal lining of the abdominal cavity, can be **localised** to one part or **generalised**, the latter **primary** or **secondary**.

A: **Localised:** Common causes are appendicitis, cholecystitis, diverticulitis, salpingitis.
Primary generalised peritonitis: bacterial infection of the peritoneal cavity without obvious focus responsible, possibly via haematogenous or lymphatic spread, or ascending infection from the female genital tract. More common in those with ascites, e.g. liver cirrhosis (SBP) or children with nephrotic syndrome.
Seconday generalised peritonitis: Peritonitis due to bacterial translocation and spread, evolving from a localised focus (see above) or nonbacterial due to spillage of bile, blood, gastric contents, e.g. perforated peptic ulcer, pancreatic secretions (a chemical peritonitis that often becomes secondarily infected).

A/R: See above.

E: Primary peritonitis is rare, usually presents in adolescent females; localised and secondary generalised peritonitis are common in surgical patients.

H: A careful history should be taken with exploration of the onset, nature, course and radiation of the abdominal pain as well as exacerbating, relieving and associated factors. Parietal pain from peritonitis is usually continuous, sharp, localised, exacerbated by movement and coughing (parietal peritoneum is supplied by somatic A-δ fibres arising from spinal nerves of T7–L2). In those with liver disease and ascites, symptoms can be vague (e.g. ↑ confusion due to encephalopathy).

E: General state should be assessed, vital signs, signs of dehydration or compromised perfusion (e.g. due to hypovolaemia, sepsis or circulatory failure).
Localised: Tenderness on examination with *involuntary guarding*: reflex contraction of overlying abdominal wall muscles; *rebound tenderness*: sudden removal of a palpating hand causes pain due to movement of the inflamed peritoneum, similarly demonstrated as percussion tenderness or pain evoked by coughing.
Generalised: Patient is usually very unwell with systemic signs of toxaemia or sepsis (e.g. fever, tachycardia). The patient lies still with shallow respiratory effort as movement exacerbates pain. The abdomen is rigid with generalised tenderness, bowel sounds are reduced or more typically absent due to paralytic ileus. Rectal examination allows direct palpation of the pelvic peritoneum usually demonstrating anterior tenderness.

P: The peritoneum consists of a single layer of flattened mesothelial cells over loose areolar tissue containing a rich network of capillaries, lymphatics, nerve endings, and immune-competent cells, particularly lymphocytes and macrophages. Secondary bacterial peritonitis is usually polymicrobial with synergistic growth of aerobic and anaerobic organisms, often arising from bowel flora. Primary peritonitis is often 'monomicrobial' (e.g. streptococcus, pneumococcus). When inflamed, the peritoneum loses its glistening appearance and becomes erythematous with production of copious serous inflammatory exudate, rich in white blood cells, protein and inflammatory mediators. The greater omentum often becomes adherent to inflamed organ, providing a barrier to spread of infection.

I: As indicated by history and clinical assessment.
Blood: FBC, U&Es, LFT, amylase, CRP, clotting, G&S or crossmatch, blood cultures, pregnancy test, ABG (looking for acidosis or respiratory failure).
Imaging: Erect CXR (for pneumoperitoneum), AXR (e.g. in bowel obstruction), USS or CT abdomen. Laparoscopy.

If ascites: Ascitic tap and cell count (diagnostic of SBP if > 250 neutrophils/ mm^3), Gram stain and culture.

M: Localised: Treatment will depend on underlying cause (e.g. appendicectomy in appendicitis), whereas other conditions may be treated with IV antibiotics (e.g. cholecystitis, salpingitis and most cases of acute diverticulitis).
Generalised: Patient is at risk of death from sepsis and shock. Needs IV fluid resuscitation and correction of volume and electrolyte imbalance (there is often severe hypovolaemia seconday to third space losses; hence fluid replacement is vital), IV antibiotics. Urinary catheter, NG tube and CVP line to monitor fluid balance. Urgent laparotomy should be performed to remove the infected or necrotic tissue, treat the cause and perform peritoneal washing with copious irrigation to remove all seropurulent exudate. An exception would be acute non-necrotising pancreatitis. Primary peritonitis is treated with antibiotics, but this diagnosis is often not apparent until after attempted operative intervention.
Spontaneous bacterial peritonitis: Medical treatment with quinolone antibiotic or cefuroxime and metronidazole combination.

C: Early: Septic shock, respiratory or multiorgan failure, paralytic ileus, wound infection, tertiary peritonitis (persistence of intra-abdominal infection), abscesses, portal pyaemia/hepatic abscesses.
Late: Incisional hernia, adhesions.

P: With appropriate treatment of the underlying cause, localised peritonitis usually resolves. Generalised peritonitis has a much higher mortality, approaching 30–50%. The concurrent development of septic shock or multiorgan dysfunction can ↑ the mortality rate to > 70%. Primary peritonitis has a good prognosis with appropriate antibiotic therapy. The overall mortality rate of patients with SBP may exceed 30% if diagnosis and treatment are delayed.

CONDITIONS

D: The formation of fibrotic plaques in the penis resulting in pain and abnormal curvature during erection.

A: Unknown.

A/R: Associated with HLA-B7, a family history of connective tissue disorders, vitamin E deficiency and 30% of patients suffer from other fibrotic conditions such as Dupuytren's contracture. DM and trauma to the penis are risk factors for disease development.

E: Relatively common, affecting 1–3% of men usually between 45 and 65 years.

H: Pain, abnormal curvature and distortion of the penis (indentation, shortening) during erection.

E: A firm plaque of tissue can be felt on the dorsal or ventral surface of the penis.

P: Slowly progressive asymmetrical fibrotic plaques develop in the tunica albuginea that surrounds the corpora carvenosa of the penis.

I: Not normally needed.
Radiographs or USS: Can identify calcified plaques.
Plaque biopsy: For rapidly progressing disease to exclude malignancy.

M: Patients are not treated surgically initially as some experience spontaneous improvement and are advised to wait for 1–2 years.
Medical: Oral vitamin E supplements and para-aminobenzoate are used. Local injections of collagenase, steroids and calcium channel blockers into the plaque have all been attempted with inconclusive effectiveness. Low-dose radiation therapy can reduce pain but has no effect on the plaque.
Surgical: Excision of the plaque and skin graft or the removal of tissue on the opposite side to the plaque to counteract the abnormal curvature (Nesbit procedure). Penile implants may be combined with the above procedures or may even be corrective alone.

C: In severe cases, erectile dysfunction may develop. Tissue atrophy may occur with some of the medical treatments. Excision of the plaque may result in partial loss of erectile function and rigidity, whereas Nesbitt procedure causes a shortening of the erect penis.

P: Good, with most patients maintaining good sexual function even without treatment.

D: A pilonidal sinus (Latin for 'nest of hair') is an abnormal epithelium-lined tract filled with hair that opens to the skin surface, most commonly in the natal cleft.

A: Proposed to be caused by shed or sheared hairs penetrating the skin and inciting an inflammatory reaction and sinus development, with intermittent negative pressure drawing in more hair and perpetuating the cycle.

A/R: Associated with hirsute individuals and those who spend a long time sitting (known as 'jeep bottom' during World War II). Certain occupations may predispose, e.g. hairdressers may develop interdigital pilonidal sinus.

E: Common, affecting 0.7% young adults (male : female is 4 : 1).

H: Painful natal cleft, especially if inflamed or superimposed infection, and the patient may complain of a discharging swelling. Often a recurrent problem.

E: Presence of midline openings or pits seen between the buttocks, from which hairs may protrude. If associated infection or abscess, a tender swelling develops that may be fluctuant or discharge pus or bloodstained fluid on compression. Secondary openings may be seen on either side of the midline.

P: The sinus tract is lined with squamous epithelium and extends a variable distance into SC tissue, often with branching side channels. Hair shafts and foreign body giant cells are seen in associated granulation tissue. Tracking of bacteria leads eventually to inflammation and the formation of an SC polymicrobial abscess filled with granulation tissue, pus and hair.

I: None needed for diagnosis.
Bloods: FBC (for raised WCC), fasting glucose (for diabetes).

M: **Surgical:**
Acute pilonidal abscess: Usually requires incision and drainage (can be done under local anaesthesia if small) with removal of pus, hair and granulation tissue. The cavity is packed (e.g. with iodine-soaked dressings) and changed regularly until there is secondary closure. Antibiotic cover post-op is usually unnecessary.
Chronic pilonidal sinus: Excision under general anaesthesia with exploration, laying open and removal of tracts (may be identified by staining with methylene blue). The fibrous tissue tracts attached to the sacrococcygeal bone can be divided. Wound healing is improved if the initial incision is not in the midline (e.g. Karydakis operation). The Bascom technique involves an incision lateral to the midline for removal of the chronic abscess cavity with removal of the small midline pits using small incisions that are then closed, leaving the lateral wound open.
Prevention: Good hygiene in the area is essential; shaving is important in preventing recurrence.

C: Pain, infection, abscess, recurrence.

P: Good with drainage of pilonidal abscess. Shaving results in cure in many cases, but may be a recurring problem. Usually resolves by age of 40.

Pressure sores

D: Skin damage and ulcers caused by pressure on weightbearing areas, typically tissue over bony prominences.

A: Pressure on susceptible tissues results in impaired perfusion, ischaemia, cell death and skin breakdown.

A/R: **Extrinsic:** Pressure, shear, friction, moisture.
Intrinsic: Age, immobility, sensory impairment, incontinence, protein-calorie malnutrition (for each 10 g/L ↓ in albumin, threefold ↑ in risk).

E: Common, 3–10% of hospitalised patients and nursing home residents, with > 70% in those aged > 70 years, with annual costs estimated at £321m. in the UK.

H: Area of erythema or ulcer may be noticed by carer, less frequently the patient may complain of pain in the affected area. Predisposing factors should be ascertained. The ischaemic injury responsible may have occurred early on in a hospital stay, e.g. while on operating table, with the majority developing within the first 2 weeks.

E: Vulnerable areas are over the sacrum, coccyx, ischial tuberosities, greater trochanter malleoli and heels, also the occiput and scapulae.
Stage I: Nonblanching erythema with intact epidermis.
Stage II: Shallow ulcer involving dermis (can be a blister).
Stage III: Full thickness of dermis, extending into SC tissue.
Stage IV: Extending beyond deep fascia into tendon, bone, muscle or joint.
This system cannot be used to measure progression or healing (e.g. Stage IV ulcers do not always start and progress through Stages I, II and III).
Colonisation of wounds by bacteria is common and unavoidable; however, infection should only be diagnosed if there is associated erythema, odour, purulent exudates or systemic signs (e.g. fever).

P: When external pressure exceeds capillary filling pressure (32 mmHg), tissue perfusion is impaired resulting in ischaemia, acidosis and waste product accumulation. Early signs of tissue damage occur in the dermis with nonblanching erythema indicating perivascular haemorrhage from capillaries. With time there is cell death and tissue necrosis in the dermis, SC tissues and then the epidermis.

I: Wound swab, FBC, blood cultures if infection suspected.
Plain radiographs, bone or [67]Gallium scans, MRI or needle bone biopsy if underlying osteomyelitis is suspected.

M: **Prevention** is the key: Risk assessment (e.g. Waterlow scores), assessing nutritional status, avoiding excessive bed rest.
Pressure reduction: Turning the patient every 2 h. Avoiding pressure on vulnerable sites, especially sacrum, trochanters and heels, pressure-reducing devices (static or dynamic) such as foam or air mattresses that distribute the pressure between the patient and the bed.
Wound management: Pressure reduction. Assessing severity and optimising wound environment to promote granulation and re-epithelialisation, debridement of necrotic tissue. Use of appropriate dressings (e.g. hydrocolloid, hydrogel or alginates). Prevention and treatment of infection, attention to nutrition (vitamin C, zinc supplementation in those who are deficient).
Surgical: Restricted to Stage III or IV ulcers. Debridement of necrotic material and reconstruction of affected area with myocutaneous flaps (have a high complication rate, hence attention to pre-op optimisation and post-op care are vital).

C: Infection (e.g. cellulitis or osteomyelitis), chronic ulceration, tendency to recur.

P: Pressure ulcers are difficult to heal, Stage II may take several weeks of care, while only ⅓ of Stage IV have healed after 6 months; hence, prevention is vital.

D: Primary malignant neoplasm of the prostate gland.

A: Unknown.

A/R: Age is the biggest risk factor. Race (Afro-Carribean > Caucasian, and the former tend to present at a younger age with more aggressive disease). Geographic distribution (higher in North America, Europe; low in Far East). Family history (a gene on chromosome 1 implicated). Dietary factors (high fat, meat and alcohol consumption associated, ↓ with soy). Occupational exposure to cadmium and ↑ sexual partners suggested but not proven.

E: Common, second most common cause of male cancer deaths. Incidence in the West of 50–70/100 000. Microfoci of cancer are found in 80% of men over 80 on autopsy.

H: Often asymptomatic and detected on PSA testing.
Lower urinary tract obstruction: Frequency, hesitancy, poor stream, nocturia and terminal dribble.
Metastatic spread: Bone pain or spinal cord compression from bone metastases.
General symptoms of malignancy (malaise, anorexia and weight loss).
Paraneoplastic syndromes (e.g. hypercalcaemia).

E: Asymmetrical hard nodular prostate gland with loss of the midline sulcus on rectal examination.

I: **Bloods:** FBC, U&Es, PSA, acid phosphatase, LFT, bone profile.
Prostate-specific antigen: Debatable if this is a suitable tool for screening, as values are age-related and may be ↑ in benign prostatic hyperplasia, prostatitis, following catheterisation. Refinements to improve sensitivity include PSA velocity (rate of change), PSA density and free and complex PSA values.
CT/MRI scan: Assesses extent of local invasion and lymph node involvement.
TRUS and needle biopsy: For histological diagnosis.
Isotope bone scan: For bone metastases.

P: **Macro:** 70% of prostate carcinoma develops from the peripheral prostatic gland, 10% from the paraurethral tissue and 20% from the transition zone. 85% are diffuse multifocal tumours.
Micro: Adenocarcinoma (95%) with a variable degree of differentiation.
Gleason score: Grading based on histology, two scores are given based on predominant appearance, with maximum score of $5 + 5$ (10).
Spread: Local growth into seminal vesicles, bladder and rectum; lymphatic spread to iliac and para-aortic nodes; blood-borne spread most commonly to bone (especially to the spine) as well as lung or liver.
Staging: TNM system: T1a: incidental < 5% on TURP; T1b: incidental > 5% on TURP; T1c: identified on needle biopsy. T2: confined to prostate (a: one lobe, b: both lobes). T3: extending through capsule. T4: fixed tumour invading adjacent structures other than seminal vesicles. N1: regional lymph nodes involved. M: metastases.

M: **Multidisciplinary discussion:** On tumour staging and optimal treatment modality considering patients age, comorbidity and wishes.
Active surveillance: Watchful waiting and PSA monitoring may be appropriate in the more elderly, asymptomatic patient with small, well-differentiated tumours.
Medical hormone therapy: Androgen ablation SC LHRH analogues, e.g. goserelin combined initially with anti-androgen (cyproterone acetate) to prevent testosterone flare. Other therapies include anti-androgens: nonsteroidal, e.g. bicalutamide, flutamide or steroidal.

CONDITIONS

CONDITIONS

Surgical: Radical prostatectomy in tumours localised to the gland. This can be done either by retropubic (which allows pelvic lymph node sampling) or perineal approaches. Androgen ablation by bilateral orchidectomy.

Radiological: Adjuvant radiotherapy if the surgical excision margins are inadequate or there is lymph node involvement to tumours confined to the pelvis. Brachytherapy can also be used. Neoadjuvant hormone treatment has been shown to be effective prior to external beam radiotherapy to large but localised tumours. Palliative radiotherapy can be used for bone pain and neurological complications

C: **Disease:** Obstructive hydronephrosis, hypercalcaemia, spinal cord compression.
From surgery: Impotence, urinary incontinence, urethral stricture.
From radiotherapy: Bowel and bladder damage.
From hormone therapy: Androgen deficiency can cause impotence, ↓ libido, gynaecomastia, hot flushes, osteoporosis. Tumour hormone escape can result from tumours that evolve cell lineage dominance, which is independent of anti-androgen therapy and is very difficult to manage.

P: Untreated 5-year survival of 80%; radical treatment has a 10-year survival of more than 80%. Metastatic disease has a median survival of 18–24 months.

D: Occlusion of pulmonary vessels, most commonly by a thrombus that has travelled to the vascular system from another site.

A: Thrombus ($>95\%$ originating from DVT of the lower limbs and rarely from right atrium in patients with atrial fibrillation). Other agents that can embolise to pulmonary vessels include amniotic fluid embolus, air embolus, fat emboli, tumour emboli and mycotic emboli from right-sided endocarditis.

A/R: Risk factors for DVT (Virchow's triad*), e.g. surgical patients, immobility, obesity, OCP, heart failure, malignancy.

E: Relatively common, especially in hospitalised patients, they occur in 10–20% of those with a confirmed proximal DVT.

H: Depends on the size and site of the pulmonary embolus:
Small: May be asymptomatic.
Moderate: Sudden onset dyspnoea, cough, haemoptysis and pleuritic chest pain.
Large (or proximal): All of the above plus severe central pleuritic chest pain, shock, collapse, acute right heart failure or sudden death.
Multiple small recurrent: Symptoms of pulmonary hypertension.

E: **Small:** Signs may be absent. Low-grade pyrexia and tachycardia. Low saturation O_2.
Moderate: Tachypnoea, tachycardia (may be atrial fibrillation), pleural rub, low saturation O_2 (despite oxygen), signs of DVT (see Deep vein thrombosis).
Massive PE: Shock, cyanosis, signs of right heart strain ($\uparrow$ JVP, left parasternal heave, accentuated S_2).
Multiple recurrent PE: Signs of pulmonary hypertension and right heart failure.

P: **Moderate PE:** Occlusion of pulmonary artery branches causes pulmonary infarction and a peripheral wedge-shaped haemorrhagic area. There may be a coexisting compromised collateral bronchial artery circulation.
Massive PE: Large emboli may wedge at the pulmonary artery bifurcation (saddle embolus).

I: **Bloods:** ABG, D-dimer tests (for cross-linked fibrin degradation products released into the circulation following fibrin breakdown; it is not very specific, especially if post-surgical but negative result makes PE very unlikely); thrombophilia screen if indicated prior to starting anticoagulation.
ECG: May be normal or more commonly show a tachycardia, right axis deviation or RBBB. Classical S_I, Q_{III}, T_{III} pattern is relatively uncommon.
CXR: Often normal. May show a wedge-shaped peripheral opacity, pulmonary oligaemia ($\downarrow$ vascular markings), linear atelectasis or a small pleural effusion. Mainly to exclude other differential diagnoses.
Ventilation-perfusion scan: Administration of IV ^{99m}Tc macro-aggregated albumin and inhalation of ^{81}krypton gas. This identifies any areas of ventilation and perfusion mismatch that would indicate infarcted lung. May be difficult to interpret if there is coexisting lung disease.
Spiral CT pulmonary angiogram: Non-invasive. Poor sensitivity for small emboli, but very sensitive for medium to large emboli. Investigation of choice if there is underlying lung disease.
Pulmonary angiography: Gold standard, but invasive. May be done prior to surgery for massive emboli.
Doppler USS of the lower limb: To examine for venous thrombosis.
Echocardiogram: May show thrombus in heart or pulmonary artery.

M: **Primary prevention:** Graduated pressure stockings (TEDs) and heparin prophylaxis in those at risk (e.g. undergoing surgery). Early mobilisation and adequate hydration post surgery.

CONDITIONS

CONDITIONS

If haemodynamically stable: O_2, anticoagulation with heparin or LMW heparin, changing to oral warfarin therapy (INR 2–3) for a minimum of 3 months. Analgesics for pain.

If haemodynamically unstable: Resuscitate, give oxygen, IV fluid resuscitation, thrombolysis with tPA has been used. Analgesia, followed by prevention of further thrombi (see above).

Surgical or radiological: Embolectomy (when thrombolysis is contraindicated). IVC filters (Greenfield filter) may be inserted when there are recurrent pulmonary emboli despite adequate anticoagulation or when anticoagulation is contraindicated.

C: Death, pulmonary infarction, pulmonary hypertension, right heart failure (cor pulmonale).

P: 30% untreated mortality, but only 8% with treatment (due to recurrent emboli or underlying disease). Patients have ↑ risk of future thromboembolic disease.

*Virchow's triad comprises disorders of blood flow (e.g. venous stasis), disorders of the vessel wall (e.g. endothelial injury) and disorders of blood composition (e.g. thrombophilia).

D: Thickening of the circular muscle of the pylorus in infants resulting in gastric outflow obstruction.

A: Unknown factors appear to cause an imbalance between gastric and pyloric muscle contractions leading to hypertrophy and hyperplasia of the pyloric smooth muscle.

A/R: Family history, with inheritance more often from the maternal side and in firstborns.

E: Incidence $\sim$3/1000, male:female is 4:1, typically at $\sim$6 weeks of age but can occur up to 7 months in premature babies.

H: Baby develops forceful 'projectile' vomiting of milk, not bilious but may be blood-stained due to associated oesophagitis. Although initially well and appearing hungry, the baby with time becomes lethargic and dehydrated.

E: Baby may appear well, or underweight and show signs of dehydration (5–15% body weight, sunken fontanelles, dry mucous membranes, poor skin turgor). Abdominal examination can show gastric peristaltic waves from the left to right upper quadrant. The hypertrophied pylorus may be felt as a pyloric 'tumour', an olive-sized firm lump in the right of the epigastrium.

P: **Macro:** The pylorus thickens and enlarges to form a firm oval mass, often with associated gastric enlargement and gastritis or oesophagitis.
Micro: There is hypertrophy and hyperplasia of the smooth muscle.

I: **Bloods:** U&Es, capillary gases to determine metabolic derangement (metabolic alkalosis with $\downarrow$ K^+ and $\downarrow$ Cl^-, the latter giving an indication of the severity of dehydration.
Imaging: Ultrasound demonstrates the thickened pylorus muscle and narrowed pyloric canal (wall thickness $>$ 4 mm, total diameter $>$ 10 mm, length $>$ 18 mm).

M: **General:** Correction of biochemical abnormalities and rehydration is carried out with IV fluids prior to any surgery (if not, there is a risk of apnoea post anaesthesia because of loss of respiratory drive from both $\downarrow$ H^+ due to alkalosis and $\downarrow$ CO_2 due to ventilation). An NG tube is inserted to prevent aspiration of gastric contents and fluid and electrolyte imbalance are corrected over at least 24 h.
Surgical: Ramstedt's pyloromyotomy is the definitive procedure undertaken usually in a specialist paediatric surgical department. Through the initial incision (e.g. midline rectus splitting incision) the pylorus is identified, the serosa cut by knife or diathermy and the circular muscle then split along the anterior wall with a mosquito forceps down to the mucosa. The stomach is then filled with air to ensure that the mucosa has not been perforated (if this is the case, the defect should be sutured and an omental patch sutured over the mucosa). Post-op, the child can be fed within a few hours of surgery, but if the mucosa has been breached, this is withheld for 24 h and antibiotics are given.

C: Malnutrition, dehydration, hypochloraemic hypokalaemic metabolic alkalosis, gastritis and oesophagitis, aspiration and respiratory distress syndrome.
Of surgery: mucosal perforation, wound infection, incisional hernia. Post surgery, persistent vomiting is seen in $\sim$10% but usually settles (may be due to reflux disease).

P: Usually excellent. Morbidity $<$ 3%, mortality $<$ 0.5% in those undergoing surgery.

CONDITIONS

Rectal prolapse

D: The abnormal protrusion of the full thickness (or only the mucosal layer) of rectum through the anus.

A: Straining in association with abnormal rectal anatomy or physiology (deep pouch of Douglas, pelvic floor weakness, poor fixation of rectum to sacrum and ↓ anal sphincter pressure).

A/R: Constipation and causes of ↑ straining. In children it is associated with cystic fibrosis. Previous trauma to the anus or pelvic area, neurological conditions, e.g. cauda equine syndrome, multiple sclerosis are risk factors.

E: Relatively common, affecting 5–10/1000. Two peaks: in children <3 years (male = female); and the elderly (female : male is 6 : 1).

H: Protruding anal mass, initially related to defecation, may require digital replacement. Constipation, faecal incontinence, passing mucus or bleeding PR associated. May present as an emergency with irreducible or strangulated prolapse.

E: The prolapse may be seen on straining, with severity varying from protruding rectal mucosa to frank rectal prolapse (if >5 cm, invariably a complete prolapse).
May be ulcerated or may show necrosis if vascular supply is compromised.
↓ Anal sphincter tone.

P: **Incomplete prolapse:** When the prolapse only involves the mucosa, is seen in both children and adults and is associated with excessive straining, constipation and haemorrhoids.
Complete prolapse: Involves the entire rectal wall and intervening peritoneal sac occurring mainly in adults being associated with weak pelvic and anal musculature. Associated with a floppy and redundant sigmoid colon. Disease starts with prolapse only on defecation with spontaneous retraction, which can eventually progress to full prolapse.

I: **Imaging:** Proctosigmoidoscopy, defecating proctogram or barium enema.
Other: Anal sphincter manometry, pudendal nerve studies.
Sweat chloride test: In children, as ~10% will have cystic fibrosis.

M: **Initial:** Gentle digital pressure to reduce the prolapse.
Conservative: Treatment for constipation with bulk laxatives. In children, a high-fibre diet and constipation treatment is usually sufficient.
Surgical: *Incomplete prolapse:* Submucosal injection sclerotherapy with phenol-in-oil, mucosal banding or haemorrhoidectomy are suitable treatments. *Complete prolapse:* Operative repair using laparoscopic, abdominal or perineal approaches, e.g. Ripstein rectopexy: the rectum is mobilised and secured to the sacrum with nonabsorbable sutures; Delorme's procedure: excision of the rectal mucosa with plication of the underlying rectal muscle. Anal sphincter repair may be required in some cases.
Emergency: Acute prolapse may be manually reduced after adequate analgesia; if the bowel is gangrenous, excision by rectosigmoidectomy.

C: Mucosal ulceration, rectal bleeding and incontinence. Rarely, strangulation and necrosis of prolapsed bowel.

P: Spontaneous resolution usually occurs in children. Generally good in adults with appropriate treatment though there is a 15% recurrence rate.

D: Stenosis of the renal artery that can result in hypertension and renal failure.

A: Major causes are atherosclerosis and fibromuscular dysplasia (younger ages).

A/R: Atherosclerotic form is commonly associated with peripheral vascular disease, aortic aneurysm and coronary artery disease. Rarer associations of RAS are neurofibromatosis, Marfan's syndrome, Takayasu's disease, systemic vasculitis, idiopathic hypercalcaemia, renal artery aneurysms.

E: Prevalence is unknown but believed to account for 1–5% of all hypertension; fibromuscular dysplasia occurs mainly in women with hypertension at < 45 years.

H: Suspect if history of hypertension in those < 50 years, refractory to treatment, or presenting with accelerated hypertension and renal function deterioration after starting an ACE inhibitor, or history of flash pulmonary oedema.

E: Signs of hypertension (e.g. vascular changes on fundoscopy).
Renal failure.
An upper abdominal bruit may be heard over the stenosed artery.

P: Atherosclerotic RAS is usually due to widespread aortic disease involving the renal artery ostia, can be classified as osteal or non-osteal. Fibromuscular dysplasia (aetiology unknown) results in focal stenosis (see Fig. 26a) that may be associated with micro-aneurysms in the mid and distal renal arteries (resembling string of beads on angiography). Renal hypoperfusion stimulates the renin-angiotensin system leading to ↑ circulating angiotensin II and aldosterone, increasing BP, which in turn, with time, causes fibrosis, glomerosclerosis and renal failure.

I: **Non-invasive:** Duplex USG (technically demanding and difficult if obese). Ultrasound measurement of kidney size (predicts outcome after revascularisation, kidneys < 8 cm are unlikely to improve). MRA or CT angiography.
Invasive: Digital subtraction angiography.
Renal scintigraphy: With ^{99m}Tc-DTPA (excreted by glomerular filtration) or ^{99m}Tc-MAG$_3$ (excreted by tubules), the addition of an ACE inhibitor (captopril renography) causes delayed clearance by the affected kidney (may not be helpful if bilateral RAS).

M: **Medical:** Pharmacological control of hypertension. In atherosclerotic cases, medical treatment is often preferred together with modulation of other cardiovascular risk factors. Avoidance of ACE inhibitors and other nephrotoxic agents.
Intervention: In cases of uncontrolled hypertension, progressive renal failure, flash pulmonary oedema, stenoses > 60%.
Angioplasty +/− stenting: Treatment of choice for fibromuscular dysplasia, less effective in atherosclerotic cases (see Fig. 26b). .
Surgical revascularisation: Several approaches are used, e.g. aortorenal bypass using saphenous vein or synthetic grafts (PTFE or Dacron), aortic replacement and renal reconstruction, endarterectomy of atherosclerotic RAS, extra-anatomical bypass (hepatorenal on right, splenorenal on left).

C: Drug-refractory hypertension, renal failure.
Of angioplasty: Restenosis (occurs in up to 20%), rarely renal artery rupture or thrombotic occlusion may require emergency surgery (with high mortality ∼ 40%).

P: Untreated hypertension will progress to renal failure. With intervention 50–70% will have improvement in BP and renal function. Curative in 15%.

CONDITIONS

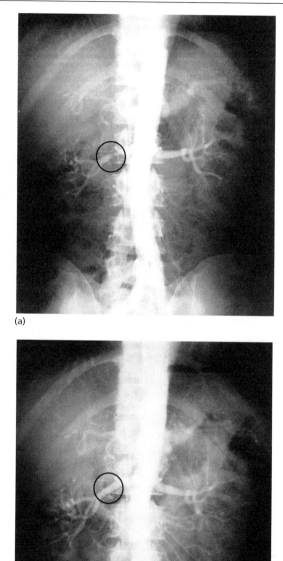

(a)

(b)

Fig. 26 (a) Renal artery stenosis (right renal artery); (b) Same individual post right renal artery angioplasty.

D: Primary malignancies of the kidney.

A: Renal clear cell carcinomas (80%) or papillary carcinomas (10%) are derived from proximal tubular cells of unknown aetiology. 10% are transitional cell carcinomas that occur in the renal pelvis (see *Bladder tumours*).

A/R: Associated with inherited conditions: von Hippel-Lindau disease, tuberous sclerosis, polycystic kidneys and familial RCC. Also associated with smoking and chronic dialysis.
RCC can be associated with abnormal LFT in the absence of liver metastases, a phenomenon known as Stauffer's syndrome.

E: Uncommon ($\sim$3% of all adult malignancies). Male:female is 2:1. Peak incidence in 40–60 years.

H: **Renal cell carcinomas:** Usually present late (being asymptomatic in 90%). Classic triad of haematuria, flank pain and abdominal mass (only 10% patients).
Transitional cell carcinomas: Usually present earlier with haematuria.
Systemic signs of malignancy: Weight loss, malaise, paraneoplastic syndromes: pyrexia of unknown origin, symptoms of hypercalcaemia or polycythaemia.

E: Palpable renal mass.
Hypertension, plethora or anaemia.
A left-sided tumour extending into the left renal vein can obstruct the left testicular vein causing a left-sided varicocoele.

P: **Robson staging:**
Stage 1: Confined to renal parenchyma.
Stage 2: Extends to adrenal glands and perinephric fat.
Stage 3: Involves local vessels or nodes.
Stage 4: Spreads to adjacent or distant organs.
Renal cell carcinomas: Macro: Arise from any portion of the kidney (usually the poles), appearing as spherical masses composed of yellow-white tissue that may have necrosis, haemorrhage and calcification.
Micro: 90% adenocarcinomas with small nuclei and abundant clear cytoplasm, other granular cells, occasionally sarcomatoid. Spread is often along the renal vein, with tumour emboli to the lungs. Metastasis is also to lymph nodes, bones, liver and skin.
I: Urine: Dipstick (to detect haematuria), cytology.
Blood: FBC, U&Es, Ca^{2+}, LFT, $\uparrow$ ESR in 75%.
Imaging: Ultrasound (abdominal): Most useful first-line investigation. Can distinguish between solid masses and cystic structures. KUB film and IVU are limited, being only able to detect large lesions that change the renal contour or compress the ureters. CT scans with contrast or MRI scans are more sensitive and also allow staging. Bone scan.

M: **Surgical:** Transabdominal or loin radical nephrectomy is the standard treatment with resection of perinephric fat, Gerota's fascia and ipsilateral adrenal gland. Partial nephrectomy ('nephron-sparing') may be appropriate to some patients.
Radiotherapy and chemotherapy: RCC is notoriously resistant to chemotherapeutic agents; radiotherapy may be used for metastatic lesions.
Immunotherapy: Interleukin-2 and γ-interferon have limited response rates (15–20%).

C: **Renal cell carcinomas:** Distant metastases (50% affect the lung, 33% the bone). Local invasion (e.g. IVC obstruction, invasion of perinephric fat). Local haemorrhage, clot colic. Paraneoplastic syndromes are present in 30%.
Transitional cell carcinomas: Obstruction of urinary outflow, hydronephrosis.

P: Depends on type and stage of tumour. Following resection of localised disease 5-year survival is 70–80%, with nodal extension and metastases 30% and < 10% respectively.

CONDITIONS

PROCEDURES

I: **Elective:** For end-stage renal failure requiring dialysis or predicted to require dialysis within 6–12 months. Most common causes are diabetic nephropathy, chronic glomerulonephritis, reflux nephropathy, hypertensive nephrosclerosis, polycystic kidney disease, renal vascular disease.

End-stage renal failure occurs in 8–12/100 000 per year, with over 5000 on the waiting list for transplant and ~ 1600 transplants performed annually in the UK.

A: The donor kidney is implanted heterotopically (i.e. in a different location to the native kidney) retroperitoneally in the iliac fossa. Renal vessels are anastomosed to the external iliac vessels, or sometimes in children to the aorta and IVC. The ureter is anastomosed to the bladder. Left kidneys are generally less difficult to transplant due to the longer associated vein and artery. Native kidneys are usually left in situ unless at risk of causing recurrent sepsis, or in the case of large polycystic kidneys, impinging into the iliac fossa.

I: **Cardiovascular:** Ischaemic heart disease is very common in patients on dialysis; hence should be assessed (e.g. ECG, echocardiography, perfusion studies or angiography).

Infection: Pre-op, it is important to assess the patient for any risk of infection, especially UTI and should be screened for dental problems. HIV infection is a contraindication because of the poor prognosis on immunosuppression.

Live related donors: Requires a thorough medical and psychological assessment. They should not have any significant medical problems and the function and anatomy of their kidneys are delineated.

Tissue typing: Better matching of major histocompatibility loci class II DR > I B > I A results in improved outcome. HLA typing is carried out on patients on the waiting list and also on lymphocytes from the donor lymph node or spleen. Identical or 'favorable' matches are identified, and a national organ-sharing network enables rapid identification of the most suitable recipient. Donor kidneys must be blood group compatible and recipients are screened for anti-HLA antibodies that would result in hyperacute rejection.

P: **Donor organs:** Only ~ 20% of patients (UK) have suitable living donors; the remainder of organs are from cadaveric donors (e.g. heart-beating brainstem death). Due to the shortage of organs, non-heart-beating donors are also increasing. Consent from next of kin is obtained in all cases. Donors should have good renal function, be free of systemic infection or malignancy (except for primary brain tumours) and be screened for hepatitis and HIV.

Organ retrieval: The kidneys are harvested as part of a multi-organ retrieval, minimising warm ischaemia time, perfusing the kidneys in situ with cold preservative solution (Marshall or University of Wisconsin solution). To avoid damage, the kidney is removed with perinephric fat in situ. Preservation times should be minimised but up to 24 h is tolerated; any longer can result in higher short- and long-term failure rates.

Recipient operation: An oblique lower abdominal incision is used with an extraperitoneal approach that allows access to the iliac vessels and bladder. The renal vein is anastomosed to the external iliac vein, then the end-to-side arterial anastomosis is created, often with a patch of donor aorta (Carrel patch). If the donor artery does not have a patch (e.g. a living donor kidney), the artery may be anastomosed end-to-end to the recipient internal iliac artery (see Fig. 27). A ureteroneocystostomy is then created, implanting the ureter directly or through a submucosal tunnel to minimise reflux (e.g. modified Leadbetter–Politano technique). Sometimes a double J-stent is placed. An indwelling catheter is left for a few days to allow healing of the bladder incision. Antibiotic prophylaxis is routine. Post-op, careful attention must be placed on fluid balance.

Immunosuppression: Using cyclosporin, tacrolimus (calcineurin inhibitors), azathioprine, mycophenolate and steroids. Deterioration in renal function should be investigated by ultrasound, Doppler or biopsy.

PROCEDURES

C: **Impaired graft function:** Early oliguria or polyuria is common. Delayed graft function that may be due to acute tubular necrosis is also common (20–30%).

Vascular (1–5%): Haemorrhage, renal artery thrombosis, renal vein thrombosis (sudden pain and swelling), RAS, either early (due to kinking of artery) or late due to atherosclerosis.

Urological (2–10%): Bladder leak, ureteric leak, calyceal leak (rare), ureteric stenosis (treated by ureteroplasty and stent or open surgical intervention) or reflux.

Lymphocoeles: due to disruption of lymphatics (1–6% of transplants), managed by percutaneous drainage or marsupialisation into peritoneum.

Infection: *Early*: Bacterial infections.

Later: Opportunistic infections, e.g. CMV (typically a few weeks post transplant and presents with fever, neutropaenia, thrombocytopaenia and deranged LFT, treated by gancyclovir), also HSV, *Pneumocystis*, *Candida*

Rejection: *Hyperacute*: Due to preformed antibodies. Pre-transplant cross-matching should prevent this from occurring.

Acute: Most common type (up to 40%). Due to T cells attacking the graft (diagnosed on derangement of renal function, hypertension and renal biopsy) and treated by steroid boluses or antibody treatment (antithymocyte globulin).

Chronic: Late cause of renal deterioration with gradual reduction of renal function, proteinuria and hypertension. Resistant to most therapies and eventually graft loss will occur.

Immunosuppression: Drug effects, infections, post transplant malignancies, e.g. ↑ risk of skin cancers (squamous cell carcinoma, occur at an earlier age and are more aggressive), lymphomas (2% of renal transplant patients) and Kaposi's sarcoma.

P: Patient survival > 90% at 1 year, > 80% at 5 years. Overall graft survival 85% (cadaveric donor) and 90–95% (living donor) at 12 months with a loss of 3–5% of grafts per year after this. Cardiovascular complications are the most common cause of death post transplant.

PROCEDURES

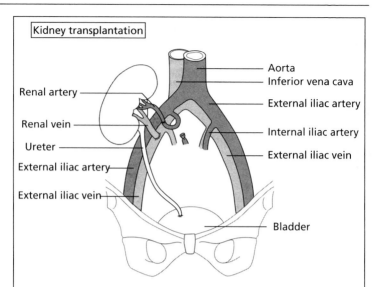

Kidney transplantation

(a) The renal artery is anastomosed (end to end) to the internal iliac artery. The renal vein is anastomosed (end to side) to the external iliac vein. The ureter is implanted in the dome of the bladder

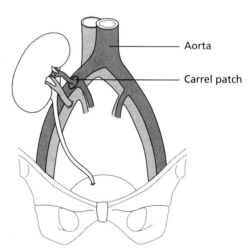

(b) The renal artery on a carrel patch is anastomosed (end to side) to the external iliac artery. Carrel patch comes from non-living (brain stem dead) donor's aorta

Fig. 27

D: Separation of the inner layers of the retina from the underlying retinal pigment epithelium (RPE) and choroid.

A: Proliferative diabetic retinopathy, sickle-cell disease, advanced retinopathy of prematurity and penetrating trauma give rise to tractional and or rhegmatogenous retinal detachment. Tumour growth and inflammation give rise to exudative or serous detachments.

A/R: Associated with myopia, aphakia, pseudophakia, i.e. cataract removal with lens implant, trauma (including previous ocular surgery), congenital malformations, metabolic disorders, vascular disease, vitreous disease or degeneration.

E: Retinal detachment usually occurs in persons aged 40–70 years.

H: Initial symptoms include the sensation of a flashing light (photopsia) accompanied by a shower of floaters. A wavy distortion of objects (metamorphopsia) may occur if the retina is involved.
Over time, the patient may notice a shadow in the peripheral visual field, which, if ignored, may rapidly involve the entire visual field.

E: Examine closely the visual acuity, visual field, pupil reaction and fundus. Indirect ophthalmoscopy is required.

P: Separation of the sensory retina from the underlying RPE occurs by the following three basic mechanisms: a break in the retina (i.e. rhegmatogenous); traction from fibrous membranes on the surface of the retina; or exudation of material into the subretinal space.

I: Imaging techniques, such as orbital films, CT scans, or MRI, are not necessary to diagnose retinal detachment, but they may be necessary to detect intraocular foreign bodies and tumours. If the retina cannot be visualised because of corneal changes or cataracts, USG is necessary.

M: **Surgical:** The repair technique is dependent on the type, location and size of the detachment. In scleral buckling a silicone band indents the eye to approximate the retina and RPE. Intraocular repair with vitrectomy may be necessary in complicated tractional and exudative detachments.
Other nonsurgical procedures: The use of intraocular gas to tamponade the detachment, laser therapy and cryotherapy.

C: Loss of vision and blindness.

P: Ultimate outcome depends upon the time, type of retinal detachment and whether the macula is involved. Prognosis is related inversely to the degree of macular involvement and the length of time the retina has been off. 15% of people with retinal detachments in one eye develop detachment in the other eye.

CONDITIONS

CONDITIONS

D: Tumours arising in either the major (parotid, submandibular, sublingual) or minor salivary glands, characterised by a diversity of histological subtypes.

A: Unknown. 80% arise in the parotid (20% malignant); 15% in the submandibular (30–50% malignant); and 15% in the minor salivary glands (>60% malignant). Sublingual gland tumours are rare (0.3%, but nearly all malignant).

A/R: Warthin's tumour is associated with smoking (8× ↑ risk), others with radiation exposure.

E: Relatively rare, most occur in adults (most common in children is haemangioma). Pleomorphic adenoma: mean age 42 years, Warthin's tumour: mean age 60 years (male > female), acinic cell carcinoma: affects women in fifties, squamous carcinomas: men in seventies.

H: A swelling, usually slow-growing and painless.
Pain is more likely if the tumour is malignant.
In locally advanced cases, induration or ulceration of overlying skin or mucosa.

E: The swelling should be examined with attention to evidence of fixation.
Inspection of the oral cavity should be performed as deep lobe parotid tumours may enlarge into the parapharangeal space, visualised as a mass lateral to the tonsil that may displace it medially or the palate downwards.
The submandibular gland should be palpated bimanually.
Facial nerve function in parotid lesions (weakness should raise suspicion of malignancy) and evidence of regional lymphadenopathy.

P: **Benign tumours:**
Pleomorphic adenoma: 80–85% of parotid gland tumours. Epithelial or myoepithelial cells without a true capsule; hence propensity to recur after removal.
Warthin's tumour (papillary cystadenoma lymphomatosum previously known as adenolymphoma): Only parotid, 15% of neoplasms, 10% bilateral or multicentric with glandular and cystic elements with eosinophilic epithelium.
Malignant carcinomas:
Acinic cell carcinoma: Most commonly in parotid. Wide histological spectrum with lymphocytic infiltrates.
Mucoepidermoid carcinoma: Most common malignant tumour of the parotid gland, of variable malignancy, i.e. low grade to aggressive.
Adenoid cystic carcinoma (6% most common malignant carcinoma of the submandibular): Aggressive with perineural spread into the brain and potential for late metastases.
Adenocarcinoma, squamous and undifferentiated carcinomas: All aggressive.
Nonepithelial tumours (e.g. haemangiomas, lymphomas): All rare.

I: **Imaging:** Ultrasound, CT or MRI scanning are useful in delineating the mass and its relationship to surrounding structures, but cannot tell if malignant.
Tissue biopsy: FNA can be used, but cannot absolutely be relied on for histological diagnosis. Incisional or excisional biopsy of masses in major glands should be avoided because of the risk of tumour spillage.
CXR: For staging if malignancy is suspected.

M: **Surgical:** Excision is used for both benign and malignant tumours.
Parotid: Superficial (for benign or low-grade malignancies) or total parotidectomy (for higher-grade malignancies) with careful preservation of the facial nerve and its branches that run between the deep and surperficial lobes. If the nerve is involved, sacrifice and immediate reconstruction with a nerve graft can be performed.
Submandibular: Tumours are approached by an incision in the submandibular triangle. Malignant tumours may involve the lingual or hypoglossal nerves and resection may be necessary. This results in partial loss of sensation, and

movement of the tongue should be discussed with the patient. There is also a risk of injury to the mandibular branch of the facial nerve resulting in asymmetry of the mouth/lower lip. Neck dissection is performed if lymph nodes are involved.

Carcinomas on the palate: Wide excision that may require complex reconstruction.

Radiotherapy: Adjuvant post-op radiotherapy should be given if malignant.

Chemotherapy: Not very successful, usually reserved for palliation.

C: **Of parotidectomy:** Facial nerve injury, hemorrhage, skin flap necrosis, salivary fistula, and Frey's syndrome (10–50%, aberrant regeneration of postganglionic parasympathetic nerve fibres that normally innervate the parotid to sympathetic nerves of sweat glands resulting in gustatory sweating).

Pleomorphic adenomas have a high rate of recurrence if only simple enucleation is performed due to presence of pseudopod-like extensions from the tumour.

P: Pleomorphic adenomas, if not removed slowly, enlarge and there is a risk of malignant transformation (5%). Mucoepidermoid carcinoma 5-year survival is 70% (but worse for higher-grade forms). Adenoid cystic carcinoma has a poor prognosis (because perineural invasion is difficult to eradicate and has tendency for late recurrence), 10-year survival is 40%, other carcinomas 5-year survival is $\sim$ 30%.

CONDITIONS

CONDITIONS

D: Epithelium-lined, keratinous, debris-filled cyst arising from a blocked hair follicle. More correctly known as epidermal cyst.

A: Occlusion of the pilosebaceous gland, traumatic insertion of epidermal elements into the dermis and embryonic remnants (see **P**athology).

A/R: More frequent in Gardner's syndrome.

E: Extremely common, any age.

H: Nontender slow-growing skin swelling, often multiple.
Common on hair-bearing areas of the body, especially face, scalp, trunk or scrotum.
May become red, hot and tender if superimposed inflammation or infection.

E: Smooth tethered lump with overlying skin punctum.
May express granular creamy material with an unpleasant smell.

P: Despite their name, these cysts are not derived from sebaceous glands. Sebaceous cysts result from the cystic proliferation of epidermal cells within the dermis. The source of this epidermis is often the infundibulum of the hair follicle. Inflammation is usually a foreign body, granulomatous reaction to material contained within the cysts.

I: None usually required.
Skin biopsy or FNA may rarely be necessary to rule out other differentials.

M: **Conservative:** May be left alone if not causing the patient distress.
Surgical: Excision of cyst can be carried out under local anaesthesia. Care must be taken to ensure complete removal or the cyst is liable to recur. If an abscess develops in association, it should be drained.
Medical: If there is infection, antibiotics may be given; however, definitive treatment involves excision once acute inflammation has settled.

C: Infection, abscess formation. Recurrence if excision is incomplete. Occasionally, may ulcerate and have the appearance of a skin malignancy (Cock's peculiar tumour). A sebaceous horn may develop if the discharging contents dry out and form a horn-shaped protrusion.

P: Excellent, most do not require treatment and excision is usually curative.

D: Joint inflammation due to intra-articular infection.

A: Bacteria enter the joint directly, e.g. penetrating wound, by haematogenous spread, systemic sepsis, adjacent osteomyelitis or a contaminated prosthesis. The most common causative organisms in < 3 years are *Staphylococcus aureus, Haemophilus influenzae* or coliforms, and *S. aureus* and *Neisseria gonorrhoeae* in adults.

A/R: Those with diabetes, corticosteroid use, IV drug abuse, immunocompromise or chronic joint disease (e.g. rheumatoid arthritis) are at ↑ risk of septic arthritis.

E: Incidence ~ 6/100 000, 50% of cases in children < 3 years.

H: Pain in a joint or limb, malaise, fever.
Commonly affects a single large joint; e.g. the hip in infants and children, present with a limp and refusing to weight bear. The knee is often affected in older children and adults, although it may affect any joint.

E: A red swollen joint; if a hip, the leg is held flexed and slightly externally rotated (slackens ligaments and reduces joint pressure).
Diffuse joint tenderness with severe reduction in its range of movement due to pain. If gonococcal arthritis, there may be associated skin pustules near the joint and evidence of urethral discharge.

I: **Bloods:** FBC, blood cultures, ESR, CRP.
Joint aspiration and microscopy, culture and sensitivity: Aspirate usually turbid with > 50 × 10³/ml white blood cells, 90% neutrophils, culture to identify causative organism.
Joint radiograph: Shows ↑ in joint space, soft tissue swelling and in late cases, subchondral bone destruction.
Bone scan: ↑ uptake is seen in joint region.
USS: To identify a joint effusion, may guide aspiration.

P: Bacteria in the joint incite an inflammatory response, with the release of inflammatory mediators and attraction of leucocytes into the joint. Activation of neutrophils, macrophages results in release of proteolytic enzymes, together with bacterial toxins cause damage to the articular cartilage. ↑ permeability and fluid secretion result in a joint effusion that may contribute to damage by ↑ pressure and ↓ synovial blood supply. During recovery, healing of the raw articular surfaces may result in fibrosis and bony ankylosis.

M: **Surgical:** In most cases, surgical washout of the joint should be carried out to remove pus and infected material. May be performed by arthroscopy or open procedure (arthrotomy). Sepsis in a prosthetic joint requires removal of the prosthesis before full eradication of infection is possible. **Medical:** Antibiotics initially, e.g. ceftriaxone or flucloxacillin, IV for 1–2 weeks followed by oral for an additional 4–6 weeks. Analgesics should be given and the joint should be splinted for pain reduction. Physiotherapy is provided to prevent fibrosis and maintain joint mobility.

C: Joint subluxation or dislocation, avascular necrosis of epiphysis, growth disturbance, ankylosis, joint destruction or secondary osteoarthritis.

P: Outcomes are dependent on the virulence of the organism, duration of infection prior to diagnosis, the premorbid condition of the patient and the joint affected, e.g. knees have better outcomes than ankles. With early appropriate treatment prognosis is usually good.

CONDITIONS

I: Indications for skin reconstruction are traumatic skin loss, e.g. burns, pressure sores, ulcers, post wide excision of large amounts of skin, e.g. after treatment for tumours or infections such as necrotising fasciitis, where primary closure or healing by secondary intention is not possible, such as exposed wounds that do not have a good blood supply, and would be disfiguring or take a long time with associated risks.

Grafts: A skin graft is a piece of skin taken from a donor site and moved to a recipient site. Skin grafts can either be **full thickness** (Wolfe graft) or **split thickness** (Thiersch graft). Meshing of the grafts creates a 'string-vest appearance'; this ↑ the surface area of the graft and allows for escape of serous or serosanguinous fluid. A disadvantage of split skin grafts is their tendency to contract, they are more subject to damage and their cosmetic appearance may be poor. Advantages of full thickness grafts include reduced contraction, ↑ robustness and better appearance, but there is often only a limited area that can be covered and are less reliable than split grafts.

Flaps: A flap is a block of tissue that brings its own blood supply with it. Flaps can be classified on the basis of their *blood supply, movement,* e.g. advancement or free flaps (the latter involving vascular or microvascular anastomosis), or *tissue content,* either single, e.g. cutaneous, fascial, bone, or composite, e.g. myocutaneous, fasciocutaneous. Advantages of flaps are that they can heal many defects, and healing times are usually faster than grafts. Disadvantages include the level of expertise required, and the donor site may be left with cosmetic or functional defects.

A: Skin is divided into three layers: epidermis, dermis and SC fascia (external to internal). Blood supply to the skin is derived from several horizontally oriented plexuses (two fascial plexuses and one subdermal plexus) and connected by vertical perforating vessels.

I: **Post-op:** Meticulous wound care and regular assessment of viability or signs of infection.

P: Numerous varied methodologies depending on donor and recipient site. Tissue that cannot form a bed of granulation tissue, e.g. cartilage, bone or bare tendon, will not support a skin graft but may be covered by a skin flap.

Split skin grafts: Epidermis and a portion of dermis is taken completely off a donor site and moved to a recipient site, deriving its blood supply from the recipient site. Can be subdivided into thin, medium or thick depending on how much dermis is removed. Common donor sites are thighs and buttocks. Grafts are anchored at the edges with sutures, staples or glue. Following placement of the graft a pressure dressing is applied to help avoid factors impairing skin graft, including infection, haematoma or seroma and shearing.

Full thickness skin grafts: Epidermis and dermis is taken from a donor site and moved to a recipient site, deriving its blood supply from the recipient site. Common donor sites include post-auricular, supraclavicular, lateral groin crease or medial arm, with the site being closed primarily.

Skin flaps: Block of skin and underlying tissue (e.g. fascia, muscle or bone) is moved from donor site to a recipient site, bringing its blood supply along. Various techniques are used to move a local flap including advancement, rotation and transposition.

C: Infection, haematoma, failure, flap necrosis, scarring, poor cosmesis.

I: **Trauma.**
Hereditary anaemias: For example, hereditary spherocytosis, elliptocytosis.
Autoimmune haematological diseases (usually as a second line measure): For example, idiopathic thrombocytopenia purpura, autoimmune haemolytic anaemia.
Myeloproliferative disorders: For example, myelofibrosis, lymphoma.
Others: Splenic vein thrombosis, Gaucher's disease.

A: The spleen lies posteriorly in the left upper quadrant of the abdomen close to the 9th–11th rib with its long axis lying along the shaft of the 10th rib. It is surrounded by peritoneum, which passes from hilum to the greater curvature of the stomach and to the left kidney as the gastrosplenic ligament (contains short gastric and left gastroepiploic vessels) and splenorenal ligament (contains splenic vessels and the tail of the pancreas) respectively. It also has multiple avascular ligamentous attachments (e.g. phrenosplenic and splenocolic ligaments). It is posterior to the stomach and left colic flexure; lateral to the left kidney and anterior to the left diaphragm, left costodiaphragmatic recess, left lung and 9th–11th rib.
Vascular: The splenic artery is from the coeliac trunk and its venous drainage is via the splenic vein, which runs behind the pancreas and joins the superior mesenteric vein to form the portal vein.

I: **Pre-op:** Ideally, vaccination against encapsulated organisms should be given 2 weeks pre-op, e.g. Pneumovax (*Streptococcus pneumoniae*), Hib (*Haemophilus influenzae*) and Men C (*Neisseria meningitidis*). Appropriate imaging (e.g. CT). FBC, U&Es, clotting, crossmatch. General anaesthetic assessment. Pre-op embolisation may reduce vascularity and aid surgery.
Post-op: Close monitoring of fluid balance and observations. Post-op changes on blood tests include a transient neutrophilia, ↑ number and size of platelets, nucleated red cells and target cells. Patients are prescribed prophylactic antibiotic cover (penicillin V or erythromycin) until age 15 years and should have a supply to start at first sign of a febrile illness.

P: **Incision:** An upper midline incision for rapid access is used in trauma cases, whereas normally a left oblique subcostal incision is made for elective cases.
(1) The ligaments on the convex surface of the spleen are identified and divided.
(2) The short gastric vessels that run from the spleen to the greater curvature are identified, ligated and divided.
(3) Blunt dissection is performed on the posterior attachments of the spleen to achieve complete spleen mobilisation around a pedicle of the splenic artery.
(4) The splenic vessels are dissected free as close to the hilum as possible to avoid injury to the pancreas. The splenic artery is doubly ligated first and blood is allowed to drain from the spleen.
(5) The splenic vein is then doubly ligated and both vessels are divided. The pedicle is now transected completely and the spleen is removed.
(6) The inferior surface of the diaphragm, greater curvature of the stomach and the region of the hilum are carefully inspected for haemostasis.
(7) Drains are only inserted if the tail of the pancreas is injured.
Closure: The wound is closed in three layers: the posterior rectus sheath and peritoneum are closed with a continuous suture, the anterior rectus sheath is closed with a separate continuous suture and the skin is closed with a continuous subcuticular suture, interrupted sutures or staples.

C: **Short-term:** Haemorrhage, damage to other organs, e.g. pancreas intraoperatively.
Long-term: ↑ Risk of sepsis, especially encapsulated organisms.

Splenic rupture

D: Rupture of the spleen due to upper abdominal or lower chest trauma.

A: Nonpenetrating trauma or rapid deceleration injury.

A/R: Associated with other traumatic internal organ injury such as rupture of the liver, left kidney, pancreas and diaphragm as well as rib fractures. Splenomegaly and its causes such as infectious mononucleosis, malaria and leukaemia ↑ the risk of rupture from even minor trauma.

E: Relatively common, some degree present in up to 25% of major trauma cases.

H: Substantial abdominal or lower chest trauma.
Abdominal pain that may be diffuse or localised to the left flank, and may result in referred pain to the left shoulder tip.

E: Skin bruising over the left flank.
Abdominal tenderness, guarding and rigidity, which is generalised or confined to the left flank; ↓ resonance over the left flank on percussion.
Left lower rib fractures.
Signs of shock (e.g. hypotension, tachycardia).

I: **Bloods:** FBC, U&Es, clotting and crossmatch.
Ultrasound: Focused abdominal sonographic technique to detect for fluid in the peritoneal cavity suggestive of intra-abdominal haemorrhage.
Diagnostic peritoneal lavage: Detects free intraperitoneal blood – rarely performed now.
CT scan: To identify splenic trauma as well as trauma to other organs.
CXR: May show rib fractures, diaphragmatic rupture or left pulmonary contusion.
AXR: May reveal displacement of the stomach bubble to the right and the splenic flexure of the colon downwards.

P: The spleen is a highly vascular organ; though protected under the rib cage, it is prone to blunt external trauma that can lead to quite extensive haemorrhage. There may be delayed rupture by up to several days post trauma due to the formation of a subcapsular haematoma that expands in size eventually rupturing. In splenomegaly, thinning of the capsule and a greater mass effect in decelerating trauma makes the spleen more fragile.

M: **Resuscitation:** IV access, fluids, transfusion if necessary, avoiding overinfusion (permissive hypotension may be tolerated). **Conservative:** Minor injuries or lacerations in a haemodynamically stable patient may be managed conservatively with close monitoring and regular review. **Interventional radiological techniques:** May be used to embolise a bleeding point.
Surgical: Emergency laparotomy if haemodynamically unstable or severe injury. Small tears may be treated by careful suturing, haemostatic absorbable gauze or partial resection. Splenectomy should be performed in more serious injuries and uncontrolled haemorrhage. **Post-op** immunisation against pneumococcal, meningococcal (Men C) and haemophilus organisms should be given. Antibiotic prophylaxis is given also up to the age of 15 with patients keeping a home supply of antibiotics to take at any sign of infection.

C: **From disease:** Haemorrhage, death.
From splenectomy: Haemorrhage, post-splenectomy sepsis, ↑ risk of encapsulated organism infections, thrombotic vascular event (splenic/splanchnic venous thrombosis), pancreatic injury, pancreatitis, subphrenic abscess, gastric distension, focal gastric necrosis.
From splenorrhaphy: Rebleeding or thrombosis of remaining spleen.

P: 75% mortality if untreated. With treatment, mean mortality ranges from 3% to 23%.

D: Slow-growing malignancy of the squamous cells in the epidermis.

A: The main aetiological risk factor is UV radiation from sunlight exposure. Can also develop in areas of skin damage in burns, radiation or from chronic skin disease (e.g. lupus, leukoplakia).

A/R: Exposure to carcinogens (like tar derivatives, cigarette smoke, soot, industrial oils and arsenic), radiation exposure, patients on long-term immunosuppression (e.g. transplant recipients, HIV patients).

E: Second most common cutaneous malignancy. Often occurring in middle-aged and elderly light-skinned individuals. Annual incidence is about 1/4000.

H: See **E**xamination.

E: Nonhealing, pink, ulcerated lesion with hard, indurated edges extending beyond visible superficial border. Variable appearance: ulcerated, hyperkeratotic, crusted or scaly.
Can occur on sun-exposed sites (face, temples, cheeks) or on mucous membranes.
It can often arise from long-standing lesions, e.g. solar keratoses, leg ulcers (Marjolin's ulcer).
Bowen's disease (intra-epidermal carcinoma in situ): solitary or multiple red-brown scaly patches often resembling psoriasis, dermatitis or dermatophyte infection.

P: **Micro:** The abnormal squamous epithelial cells often extend directly down into the dermis, through the basement membrane. In Bowen's disease, the basement membrane is intact.

I: **Skin biopsy:** Confirms malignancy and distinguishes it from other skin lesions.
Lymph node biopsy: Only necessary if suspicion of metastasis (e.g. on lips).

M: **Surgical:** For Bowen's disease, curettage and cryotherapy or cauterisation is sufficient to eradicate lesion. Invasive squamous cell carcinomas should be excised with wide margin and through SC fat, and histology is needed to confirm adequate clearance at margins.
Mohs' micrographic surgery: Excision with close margins and histological examination during surgery. Can be used in areas where large excisions are difficult, e.g. lips, near eyes.
Local radiotherapy: For larger lesions or if surgery is difficult. Usually results in a lighter scar, forming a depression.
Medical: Topical 5-fluorouracil for Bowen's disease or intralesional interferons if other options are difficult.
Follow-up should be arranged to check for recurrence.

C: Sun-exposed skin squamous cell carcinomas are usually local at the time of diagnosis, but 1/3 of those on lips or lingual membranes have metastasised by the time of diagnosis.

P: Good if treated appropriately.

PROCEDURES

I: A surgically created opening of the bowel or urinary tract to a body surface. Commonest types of stomas are ileostomy, colostomy and urostomy (others include gastrostomy, jejunostomy and caecostomy). Can be permanent or temporary.

Loop stomas: Often used to temporarily divert bowel contents to protect distal surgery, e.g. an ileoanal pouch, ileorectal or colorectal anastomosis, anal sphincter repair or to divert bowel content from diseased segments of bowel.

Emergency ileostomy or colostomy: Bowel trauma, perforation, obstruction, ischaemia, IBD, e.g. toxic megacolon. In a Hartmann's procedure, the diseased distal colon is resected with formation of an end colostomy and the distal end of the divided bowel is oversewn or closed.

Elective: End ileostomies may be created after a panproctocolectomy for ulcerative colitis, or for FAP, permanent colostomies are formed after abdominoperineal resection for low rectal carcinomas.

A: **Loop stomas:** Stomas where a loop of bowel is brought up to the surface. The proximal bowel is brought out as the stoma and the distal bowel is defunctioned. External inspection will reveal two openings

Ileostomies: Usually situated in the RIF. As output is irritant to the skin, the stomas are formed with a spout, projecting ~2.5 cm above the skin surface. Output is liquid and about 1–2 L/day, although it may diminish after a few weeks

Colostomies: Usually sited in the LIF, with the stoma flush to the skin. Output is intermittent and of a more solid consistency, depending on diet (although transverse colostomies have a more frequent semi-liquid output and can be more difficult to manage)

Stoma appliances: Consist of a pouch and a flange (the portion that sticks to and protects the skin around the stoma). The flange may consist of one or two pieces, the second piece being left attached to the skin for a few days when the pouch is changed. Some bags also have exit drains (e.g. for ileostomies) for liquid output. Charcoal filters can be used to reduce odour of flatus. (See Fig. 28.)

I: **Pre-op:** Bowel preparation may be required for some elective procedures. Pre-op counselling and stoma siting is vital. Stoma care nurse specialists have an important role. Stoma sites should ideally be marked pre-op, at a site where the patient can see the stoma, avoiding skinfolds, scars, bony prominences and the belt line.

Post-op: DVT prophylaxis. Patient education is vital.

P: **Skin incision:** A circular skin opening is created at the site marked for the stoma (placing a stoma through the rectus muscle minimises the chance of developing a hernia). The skin is incised, and SC tissues and muscle divided, and the peritoneum is opened (opening should accommodate two fingers).

Stoma formation: The end or loop of bowel is brought out through the opening. This should be a tension-free, untraumatised, well-vascularised part of bowel. The main incision is closed and dressed. The bowel is opened if it has previously been stapled or is a loop and the edges cleaned. The bowel is everted on itself and the mucosa is sutured to the skin. A transparent stoma bag is then applied to allow regular stoma inspection.

C: Relatively common (40% for ileostomies, 20% for colostomies), with ~15% necessitating operative correction.

Early: Necrosis: Can become evident within a few hours of surgery, due to compromise of the blood supply to the bowel during stoma formation, requires revision of stoma. Haemorrhage: A minor degree is common and rarely requires intervention.

Functional: Diarrhoea or constipation. Output from ileostomies can be of large volume liquid resulting in dehydration and electrolyte imbalances (can be managed by fluid replacement and bowel antispasmodics). Urinary tract calculi are more common in individuals with an ileostomy; hence the importance of hydration.

Mechanical: Dermatitis, leakage, prolapse or retraction, occasionally requiring refashioning, stenosis (may be possible to dilate using a dilator, otherwise refashioning, parastomal hernias, abscess or fistula).

Psychological: Many patients experience embarrassment, anxiety or body image problems.

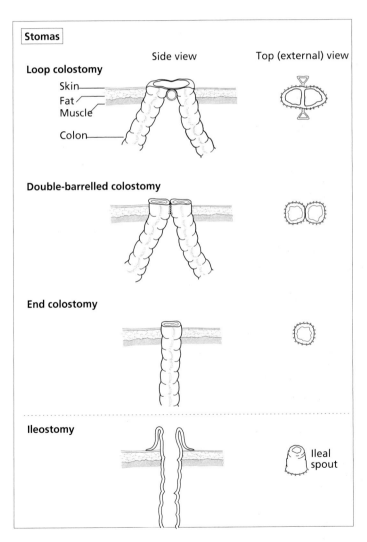

Stomas

Side view   Top (external) view

Loop colostomy
Skin
Fat
Muscle
Colon

Double-barrelled colostomy

End colostomy

Ileostomy
Ileal spout

Fig. 28

PROCEDURES

Subarachnoid haemorrhage

D: Haemorrhage into the subarachnoid space, the CSF-containing space between the arachnoid mater that lines the internal surface of the dura and pia mater that covers brain and spinal cord.

A: 85% rupture of a saccular (berry) aneurysm, 5% AVMs.
Others: Trauma, perimesencephalic haemorrhage, vertebral or carotid artery dissection with intracranial extension, mycotic aneurysms, drug abuse, e.g. cocaine.

A/R: Family history, smoking, excess alcohol intake. Saccular aneurysms are associated with polycystic kidney disease, collagen deficiency type III, Marfan's syndrome, pseudoxanthoma elasticum, Ehlers–Danlos syndrome and tuberous sclerosis.

E: Annual incidence ∼ 10/100 000. Peak age in the fifties. Female : male is 5 : 3.

H: Sudden onset severe headache, classically described 'as if hit at the back of the head'). Associated nausea, vomiting, neck stiffness, photophobia.
Confusion, collapse or ↓ level of consciousness.

E: **Meningism:** Neck stiffness, Kernig's sign (resistance or pain on knee extension when hip is flexed) due to irritation of the meninges by blood.
Glasgow Coma Scale*: Assess and regularly monitor for deterioration.
Signs of ↑ ICP: Papilloedema, IVth or IIIrd cranial nerve palsy (the latter may also be due to pressure from a posterior communicating artery aneurysm). Hypertension.
Fundoscopy: Subhyaloid haemorrhage (between retina and vitreous membrane).
Focal neurological signs: Often due to ischaemia from vasospasm and reduced brain perfusion.
Classification scale: World federation of neurological surgeons scale: Grade I GCS 15, Grade II GCS 13–14, Grade III GCS 13–14+ focal deficit, Grade IV GCS 7–12+/−focal deficit, Grade V GCS 3–6+/−focal deficit.

P: Aneurysms are abnormal localised dilatation of a blood vessel, usually seen at the sites of bifurcation of arteries in the circle of Willis. The mechanism by which the aneurysms form is controversial, usually a congenital or acquired weakness in the vessel wall. 30% lie on the anterior communicating artery, 30% on the posterior communicating artery, 20% on the middle cerebral artery and 5–10% on the bifurcation of the internal carotid artery. Multiple in 20% of patients.

I: **Bloods:** FBC, U&Es, ESR, CRP, clotting, G&S.
CT scan (noncontrast): Blood is seen as hyperdense areas in the subarachnoid space, commonly in the basal cisterns or Sylvian fissure. There may be associated hydrocephalus.
Angiography (MRI, CT or intra-arterial four-vessel): To detect the site of bleeding if the patient is a candidate for surgery or endovascular treatment. Allows simultaneous treatment.
Lumbar puncture: ↑ Opening pressure, ↑ RBC, low WCC, xanthochromia (straw-coloured CSF) due to breakdown of Hb, confirmed by spectrophotometry of CSF supernatant after centrifugation.

M: **Acute:** Maintain ABC with IV fluids to maintain cerebral perfusion (0.9% normal saline or colloid – avoid 5% dextrose as may ↑ cerebral oedema), bed rest, analgesics (paracetamol or codeine) and obtain neurosurgical review. Nimodipine (calcium channel blocker PO or IV) should be given 4-hourly to prevent vasospasm.
Interventional neuroradiology: Coiling (usually with platinum) of aneurysm.
Surgical: Clipping or wrapping of aneurysm.

CONDITIONS

AVMs: May be managed by interventional radiology, radiotherapy and/or surgery.

C: Hydrocephalus due to blood obstructing CSF flow or resorption through the arachnoid villi (25%), cerebral vasospasm (occurring about 24–72 h after haemorrhage). Major neurological deficits depending on the site of haemorrhage.

P: High mortality (> 30% in the first few days). Those with a lower GCS or neurological deficit on presentation have a worse prognosis. Significant risk of a severe rebleed in the first 2 months without treatment. Lower mortality in cases of perimesencephalic subarachnoid haemorrhage and AVMs than bleeding from aneurysms.

*The **Glasgow Coma Scale (GCS)** is a rapid measure of consciousness. Made up of three components, minimal score is 3, maximal is 15.

Eye opening	Verbal response	Motor response
Spontaneously (4)	Oriented (5)	Obeys commands (6)
To speech (3)	Confused (4)	Localising pain (5)
To pain (2)	Inappropriate (3)	Flexion to pain (4)
None (1)	Incomprehensible (2)	Abnormal flexion to pain (3)
	None (1)	Extending to pain (2)
		None (1)

CONDITIONS

Subdural haematoma

D: A subdural haematoma (SDH) is a collection of blood that develops between the surface of the brain and the dura mater. Classified depending on time of symptom onset following initial injury: **Acute:** Within 72 h. **Subacute:** 3–20 days. **Chronic:** After 3 weeks.

A: Trauma causing rapid acceleration and deceleration of the brain results in shearing forces which tear veins ('bridging veins') that travel from the dura to the cortex. Bleeding occurs between the dura and arachnoid membranes. In children, trauma is also the most common cause; however, nonaccidental injury should always be considered. Rare aetiologies include vascular malformations and malignancy.

A/R: **Acute:** Traumatic acute SDHs are often associated with underlying brain injury, e.g. cerebral contusion, subarachnoid haemorrhage, diffuse axonal injury ($>$30% of cases). **Chronic:** Older age, often associated with trivial trauma or falls, cerebral atrophy. Anticoagulant therapy or coagulopathy, e.g. renal dialysis, liver disease. Alcoholics are especially at risk as resulting symptoms may be mis-ascribed. Less commonly associated with underlying brain injury. A *subdural hygroma* (a collection of blood-tinged fluid in the subdural space) is also a risk factor.

E: **Acute:** Tend to occur in younger patients/associated with major trauma (5–25% of cases of severe head injury). More common than extradural haemorrhage.
Chronic: ↑ In elderly, studies report incidence of 1–5/100 000, male : female is 2–3 : 1.

H: **Acute:** History of trauma with head injury, patient has ↓ conscious level.
Subacute: Worsening headaches 7–14 days after trauma, altered mental status, motor weakness.
Chronic: 'The great neurological imitator' can present with headache, confusion, language difficulties, psychiatric symptoms, difficulty walking, focal weakness or hemiparesis, seizures. There may or may not be a history of fall or trauma; hence have low index of suspicion.

E: **Acute:** Reduced GCS on admission. With large haematomas resulting in midline shift, an ipsilateral fixed dilated pupil may be seen (compression of the ipsilateral IIIrd nerve parasympathetic fibres), pressure on brainstem: ↓ consciousness, contralateral hemiparesis.
Chronic: Neurological examination may be normal or there may be evidence of IIIrd nerve dysfunction, papilloedema, hemiparesis or reflex asymmetry.

P: **Acute** SDHs, if not surgically removed, slowly evolve into a liquefied clot that is slowly resorbed, especially in young adults with small haematomas.
Chronic: Blood in the subdural space evokes an inflammatory response; fibroblasts invade and form neomembranes on the inner and outer surface. Spontaneous resolution is rare and chronic SDHs have a tendency to expand (theories include osmotic gradients and recurrent bleeds from dilated fragile vessels in the outer membrane).

I: **Imaging: CT head:** Crescent- or sickle-shaped mass (see Fig. 29), concave over brain surface (an extradural is lentiform in shape), CT appearance changes with time. Acute subdurals are *hyperdense*, becoming *isodense* over 1–3 weeks (such that presence may be inferred from signs such as effacement of sulci, midline shift, ventricular compression and obliteration of basal cisterns); and chronic subdurals are *hypodense* (approaching that of CSF). MRI is said to be the modality of choice in diagnosis of bilateral subacute (isodense) SDHs.

M: **Acute:** ATLS protocol with priorities of cervical spine control and ABC. With a head injury, there is significant risk of cervical spine injury. Disability: GCS, pupillary reactivity. If signs of raised ICP, osmotic diuresis with mannitol and/or hyperventilation to reduce P_aCO_2 are used (but are both controversial). Once stabilised, CT scan head. **Conservative:** If SDH < 10 mm thickness, and midline shift < 5 mm, should be followed by imaging to ensure resolution. **Surgical:** Prompt craniotomy and evacuation for symptomatic subdurals > 10 mm, with > 5 mm midline shift (studies show better outcome if within 4 h). ICP monitoring devices may be placed and the patient cared for in ITU.

Chronic: If symptomatic, treatment is predominantly **surgical:** Burr hole craniotomy; and drainage is the most commonly used treatment. Haematomas that are not fully liquefied may require craniotomy with membranectomy (higher complication rate). Peri-operative antibiotics are given and antiepileptic medication may be used in the post-op period. *Children* with chronic SDHs: Younger children may be treated by percutaneous aspiration via an open fontanelle or if this fails, placement of a subdural to peritoneal shunt.

C: Raised ICP, cerebral oedema predisposing to secondary ischaemic brain damage, mass effect (transtentorial or uncal herniation).
Post-op: Seizures are relatively common, recurrence (5–33% for CSDHs), intracerebral haemorrhage, subdural empyema, brain abscess or meningitis, tension pneumocephalus.

P: **Acute:** Poor, primarily due to underlying brain injury (extent is the most important factor on outcome), also delay to surgery, mechanism of injury, e.g. motorcycle accidents (poor outcome). Younger patients, higher GCS, reactive pupils, without multiple contusions and those who do not develop raised ICP that is difficult to control have better outcomes.
Chronic: Generally have a better outcome than acute SDHs, reflecting lower incidence of underlying brain injury, with good outcomes in 3/4 of those treated by surgery.

Testicular malignancies

D: Malignant tumour of the testes.

A: Unknown, likely gene mutations in germ cells.

A/R: Testicular maldescent or ectopic testis ↑ risk 40×. Others are contralateral testicular tumour and atrophic testis.

E: Uncommon, 1% of male malignancies, but most common malignancy in 18–35 years. Lifetime risk 1/500.

H: Swelling or discomfort of the testes.
Backache due to para-aortic lymph node enlargement.
Respiratory symptom, shortness of breath or haemoptysis from lung metastases.

E: Painless hard testicular mass (there may be a secondary hydrocoele).
Lymphadenopathy (e.g. supraclavicular, para-aortic), signs of pleural effusion.
Gynaecomastia (resulting from tumour HCG production).

P: Main types are seminomas (50%, peak in 30–40 years) and nonseminomatous germ-cell tumours or teratomas (30%, peak in 20–30 years). Rarer types include gonadal stromal tumours (Sertoli and Leydig cell tumours) and non-Hodgkin's lymphoma.
Macro: Seminomas are pale, cream-white solid and well-circumscribed tumours. Teratomas are cystic in appearance with haemorrhagic and necrotic areas.
Micro: Seminomas contain sheets of uniform, tightly packed cells that vary from well-differentiated spermatocytes to anaplastic. Teratomas can contain tissue from yolk sac, trophoblastic and embryonal cell elements with varying differentiation, and are classified on the relative proportions.
Spread: Local spread to tunica vaginalis and along the spermatic cord; lymphatic spread to para-aortic nodes, then to mediastinal and supraclavicular nodes; blood-borne spread to lungs and liver.
Royal Marsden Hospital staging:
I – Limited to testis
II – Abdominal lymphadenopathy A: < 2 cm, B: 2–5 cm, C: > 5 cm
III – Nodal involvement above the diaphragm; A, B, C as above
IV – Liver/lung metastases

I: **Bloods:** FBC, U&Es, LFTs, tumour markers should be sent: α-fetoprotein (this indicates teratomatous elements are present) β-HCG, LDH.
Urine pregnancy test: Often wil be positive if the tumour produces ß-HCG.
CXR: Demonstrates lung metastases or pleural effusion.
Testicular ultrasound: Tumours seen within the testicle, a hydrocoele may be associated.
CT scan (abdomen, thorax): For disease staging. Of brain if extensive disease.

M: **Surgical:** Radical inguinal orchidectomy to remove the affected testis. Scrotal approach or procedures are not used as this can lead to dissemination via the scrotal lymphatics.
Following chemotherapy for teratomas, residual lymph node masses in the retroperitoneum should be considered for removal by retroperitoneal lymph node dissection as ~48% of masses > 1 cm will contain either undifferentiated or mature teratoma. If seminoma post-radiotherapy masses are observed by serial scans, most shrink and calcify over time.
Medical: Adjuvant chemotherapy is used in teratomas in Stage I disease with features that predict relapse, e.g. lymphovascular invasion or Stage II and above. The most common regimen in the UK is cycles of BEP (bleomycin, etoposide, cisplatin). Also used to treat more advanced-stage seminomas.
Radiotherapy: Adjuvant radiotherapy to para-aortic lymph nodes is standard treatment in seminomas as they are very radiosensitive. Curative to small-volume Stage II disease, but masses > 5 cm should receive chemotherapy. Teratomas are not very sensitive to radiotherapy.

Fertility preservation: Patients should be offered sperm banking prior to chemo/radiotherapy.

C: **Of disease:** Metastases causing pulmonary complications, e.g. haemoptysis, cerebral metastases may cause neurological problems.

Of treatment: Side-effects of chemotherapy: subfertility, nausea and vomiting, bone marrow depression. Bleomycin can cause rashes, pneumonitis or fibrosis – a phenomenon similar to Raynaud's; platinum agents are neuro- and nephrotoxic. With long-term survival common, secondary malignancies are becoming more common.

P: Usually good with cure rates of $>90–100\%$ in early stage disease. With >20 lung metastases, very high tumour markers, bulky mediastinal disease, or liver, bone or brain involvement, 3- year survival is $\sim70\%$.

Testicular torsion

CONDITIONS

D: A surgical emergency: twisting or torsion of the spermatic cord that results initially in venous outflow obstruction from the testicle, progressing to arterial occlusion and testicular infarction if not corrected.

A: **Intravaginal** (most common type): A high investment of the tunica vaginalis around the spermatic cord enables the testis to twist within the vaginalis.
Extravaginal (seen in neonates): When the entire testes and tunica vaginalis twist in a vertical axis on the spermatic cord (due to incomplete fixation of the gubernaculum to the scrotal wall allowing free rotation).

A/R: Imperfectly descended testes, high investment of the tunica vaginalis (bell clapper testes where the epididymis is only applied to the lower half of the testis), rarely a long epididymal mesentery predisposes to torsion.

E: Annual incidence ~ 1/4000. Most common cause of acute scrotal pain in 10–18-year-olds (intravaginal). Rarely occuring in neonates (extravaginal torsion).

H: Sudden onset severe hemiscrotal pain that may be associated with abdominal pain, nausea and vomiting. The pain may awake patient from sleep or there may be history of a similar pain that spontaneously resolved.

E: The scrotum on the affected side may be swollen and erythematous with a very tender swollen testicle lying higher than the contralateral side and may be horizontal; a thickened cord may be palpable and the epididymis may be found to lie anteriorly.
The cremasteric reflex is absent.
Testicular appendix (appendix testes, appendix epididymis, hydatid of Morgagni): There may be a visible necrotic lesion on transillumination (blue dot sign).
Differential diagnosis: Epididymo-orchitis and incarcerated inguinal hernia.

P: Twisting results in compression of the veins of the pampiniform plexus from the testis and venous congestion, with progressive ischaemia and infarction if the blood supply is not restored by detorsion.

I: In general, an acutely tender and swollen testis in a young boy or adolescent should be considered torsion until proven otherwise and urgent exploration is required. Consent should include counselling about bilateral orchidopexy and orchidectomy.
Doppler or duplex imaging of the testis: May be performed but should not delay surgery. Arterial inflow may be ↓ in cases of torsion and ↑ in epididymo-orchitis.

M: **Surgical:** Exploration of the scrotum should be performed ideally within 6 h of symptoms. A horizontal or midline raphe incision is made through the skin and dartos muscle. The tunica vaginalis is opened and the testis is delivered and inspected. Untwisting is usually carried out by rotating laterally. The testis is allowed to reperfuse, and is covered with a warm saline-soaked swab for a few minutes. This is followed by bilateral orchidopexy (fixation of testis by suturing the testes with nonabsorbable sutures to the scrotal tissues at three points of a triangle to prevent recurrence). If the testis is found to be necrotic, orchidectomy is performed.

C: Testicular infarction and atrophy if not treated promptly. If left, the testes may become infected or impair fertility by promoting formation of antisperm antibodies.

P: From onset of pain, a testicular torsion may only survive 4–6 h. With prompt exploration most cases can be salvaged.

D: An epithelium-lined cyst found along the course of descent of the thyroid gland.

A: The thyroglossal duct is a tract of embryonic mesoderm that originates between the 1st and 2nd branchial pouches, represented by the foramen caecum of the tongue. It descends to a pretracheal site during development to form the thyroid gland. The duct normally disappears in the 6th week; however, if some tissue remains at any point along its course, it may develop into a cyst.

A/R: 1–2% of cases are associated with lingual or ectopic thyroid tissue. Very rare familial variants (mostly autosomal dominant in prepubertal girls).

E: Presents in children or adolescents, mean age of presentation is 5 years (but can vary from 4 months to 70 years). 3× more common than branchial cysts.

H: A swelling or lump is noticed in the midline of the anterior neck (90%; 10% can be lateral, with 95% of these on the left side).
Mostly asymptomatic, but in 5% cases there may be tenderness or rapid enlargement due to infection.

E: Midline smooth rounded swelling, typically between the thyroid notch and hyoid bone, although sometimes found in the submental region.
Moves upwards on protrusion of the tongue and with swallowing.
Can usually be transilluminated.
Differential diagnosis: Lymph node, epidermal inclusion (dermoid) cysts, salivary duct abnormality or ectopic thyroid tissue.

P: Thryoglossal cysts can occur at any point along the thyroglossal duct path, with 75% pre-hyoid. The lining is nonkeratinising stratified squamous, columnar or cuboidal epithelium with mucoid material filling the cyst.

I: None may be necessary in a euthyroid patient.
If the cyst is suprahyoid, thyroid function tests and an isotope (^{99m}Tc) should be carried out to exclude a lingual thyroid, as its removal may render the patient hypothyroid.
Ultrasound or MRI scan: To differentiate from other structures (cysts have a high signal on T2 weighting).

M: Any acute infection is treated with antibiotics.
Surgical: Excision is carried out with the Sistrunk procedure (removal of the cyst and any duct remnant along with the central portion of the hyoid bone). Rarely, the tract may extend up to the tongue, requiring removal of a small portion of the tongue.

C: Infection is the most common complication. Thyroglossal sinus or fistula may develop after infection and spontaneous rupture, after attempted drainage or incomplete excision. Carcinoma in a thyroglossal duct cyst has rarely been described.

P: Good, but even with good technique, recurrence rates are 7–8%, more commonly following infection.

CONDITIONS

Thyroid cancer

D: Malignancy arising in the thyroid gland, types include papillary, follicular, medullary and anaplastic tumours.

A: Unknown, risk factors below.

A/R: Childhood exposure to radiation (papillary tumours). Medullary thyroid carcinomas may be familial and are associated with MEN syndrome type IIa or IIb (20% cases). Lymphoma is associated with Hashimoto's thyroiditis.

E: Incidence 2–4/100 000. Female:male is 3:1. Papillary: 20–40 years. Follicular: 40–50 years, and anaplastic tumours tend to occur in older age; both are more common in areas of endemic goitre.

H: A slow-growing thyroid/neck lump/nodule. The patient may complain of discomfort while swallowing and a hoarse voice.

E: Palpable nodules or diffuse enlargement of the thyroid. If cervical nodes are enlarged, malignancy should be suspected. The patient is usually euthyroid.

P: **Micro:** The majority are adenocarcinomas: **Papillary** (70%) tend to be multifocal, a characteristic is 'orphan Annie' pale, empty and grooved nuclei. They invade lymphatics with early spread. **Follicular** (15%) are encapsulated and undergo haematogenous spread to bone and lung. Follicular tumours cannot be diagnosed on FNAC as malignancy is based on vascular and/or capsular invasion. **Medullary** (5–10%) are well-differentiated and derive from parafollicular calcitonin-secreting C cells. **Anaplastic** carcinomas are undifferenciated pleomorphic tumours, stain for cytokeratins and are very aggresive. **Lymphomas** are rare (2.5% of extra nodal lymphomas) usually diffuse B-cell types.

I: **Blood:** TFT (if hyperthyroid, thyroid nodule is less likely to be malignant), bone profile, serum thyroglobulin (tumour marker for papillary and follicular tumours) and calcitonin (tumour marker for medullary carcinoma).
FNAC or ultrasound-guided core needle biopsy: Allows for histological diagnosis.
Excision lymph node biopsy: If there is an enlarged cervical lymph node.
Isotope scan: May be necessary if nature of thyroid lump is not known.
Staging: CT or MRI scan neck, chest, bone scan.

M: **Surgical:** Total thyroidectomy with block dissection of any affected lymph nodes. Subtotal thyroid lobectomy is possible for well-localised papillary tumours. Anaplastic tumours tend to be hard fixed masses and local debulking and tracheal compression may be the only option.
Medical: Chemotherapy: Thyroxine treatment to avoid hypothyroidism post surgery and to suppress residual tumour cells in papillary and follicular tumours. Doxorubicin chemotherapy is used in anaplastic tumours.
Radiological: ^{131}I-radioiodine treatment for papillary tumour extending beyond the capsule, recurrences and metastasis. External radiotherapy for local recurrences. Anaplastic tumours are poorly responsive.

C: **From disease:** Dysphonia, hoarseness due to recurrent laryngeal nerve involvement, airway obstruction or dysphagia.
From surgery: Haemorrhage, recurrent laryngeal nerve damage, superior laryngeal nerve paresis, tracheomalacia, laryngeal oedema, hypoparathyroidism, hypothyroidism.

P: Important factors are tumour type, size and stage. Papillary carcinomas have an overall 90% 10-year survival, best in those < 40 years with tumours < 1.5 cm; follicular have overall 85% 10-year survival; medullary have 5-year surivival of 90% (node negative) and 50% (node positive), worse in men and those aged > 50 years.
Lymphomas confined within the capsule have an 85% 5-year survival, which drops to 40% with local spread.
Anaplastic carcinomas have a very poor prognosis.

D: Severe colitis associated with segmental or total dilation of inflamed colon.

A: Most commonly a severe flare of ulcerative colitis, but also may occur in Crohn's disease, pseudomembraneous colitis and other infective colitides.

A/R: Crohn's or ulcerative colitis, *Clostridium difficile* infection, amoebiasis and other infections such as *Salmonella*.

E: May occur in 3–10% of patients with ulcerative colitis, less common in Crohn's and generally rare in infective aetiologies.

H: The patient is very unwell.
Abdominal cramps pain.
Urgency and bloody diarrhoea.
Nausea and anorexia.

E: Pyrexia, tachycardia, hypotension, dehydration.
Tender distended abdomen.
↓ or loss of bowel sounds.

P: Inflammation extends into the muscular layers of the bowel wall. There is neurogenic loss of motor tone and resulting distension of the colon and risk of perforation. Mucosal sloughing and tissue necrosis with muscle thinning is seen on histological examination. Colonic bacterial overgrowth leads on to systemic toxicity from absorption through inflamed colonic mucosa.

I: **Bloods:** FBC (WCC raised dramatically), U&Es (↓ K^+), alb (↓), CRP (very high).
Radiology: AXR or CT scan will show a dilated (> 6 cm) colon. If > 10 cm high risk of perforation, and an erect CXR should be performed to detect air under the diaphragm indicating perforation. Barium enema is contraindicated as it may perforate the bowel.

M: **Medical (conservative):** The optimal management of severe colitis is multi-disciplinary with input of gastroenterologists, surgeons and intensive care. Aggressive fluid resuscitation and high-dose IV steroids/antibiotics. If significant improvement does not follow within hours or days, other therapeutic measures, e.g. IV cyclosporine therapy and surgery must be considered. In patients with toxic megacolon, early surgical intervention is indicated.
Surgical: Total colectomy with ileostomy is the appropriate surgical treatment in most cases.

C: Perforation and peritonitis. Systemic sepsis.

P: High mortality (20–30%).

Tracheostomy

I: Most common indication is longer-term ventilatory support. Severe respiratory disease, severe neurological impairment (e.g. coma, stroke, motor neuron disease), post-pharynx or larynx surgery.

A: The trachea is a cartilaginous and membranous tube, flattened at the back. The anterior surface of the trachea is convex, and covered (superiorly to inferiorly), by the isthmus of the thyroid gland, the inferior thyroid veins, the strap muscles of the neck and the cervical fascia. Tracheal cartilage rings are incomplete posteriorly.

I: Usually done under general anaesthesia.
Pre-procedure: When possible, pre-procedure counselling is recommended.
Post-procedure: Regular sterile suction of retained secretions. Humidified gases should be used.

P: **Access:** Transverse incision midway between sternal notch and cricoid cartilage. To expose the trachea, deepen incision with blunt instrument, split and retract the strap muscles, and if necessary, divide the thyroid isthmus.
Tracheostomy: Make a longitudinal incision in the trachea (2–3 tracheal rings in length). Insert a tracheostomy tube or plug into the incision (it may be necessary to remove all other intubation at the same time (e.g. endotracheal). Inflate the balloon of the tracheostomy tube and suture edges of the wound. Secure the tracheostomy tube with tapes around the patient's neck.

C: **Short-term:** Infection (*Escherichia coli*, *Pseudomonas*), tube displacement.
Long-term: Stricture formation, tracheo-oesophageal fistula.

D: Chronic relapsing and remitting inflammatory disease of the large bowel. Together with Crohn's disease, this is known as inflammatory bowel disease.

A: Unknown. Suggested hypotheses include genetic susceptibility, immune response to bacterial or self-antigens, environmental factors, altered neutrophil function, abnormality in epithelial cell integrity.

A/R: Positive family history of IBD (∼ 15%).
Associated with ↑ serum pANCA, PSC, other autoimmune diseases.

E: Prevalence: 1/1500 (in developed world). Higher prevalence in Ashkenazi Jews. Peak onset age in 20–40 years.

H: Bloody or mucous diarrhoea (stool frequency related to severity of disease). Tenesmus and urgency.
Crampy abdominal pain before passing stool, weight loss, fever.
Symptoms of extra GI manifestations (see **C**).

E: Signs of iron deficiency anaemia, dehydration.
Clubbing.
Abdominal tenderness, tachycardia.
Blood, mucus and tenderness on PR examination.
Signs of extra GI manifestations (see **C**).

P: **Macro:** Mucosal inflammation initially involving rectum and may extend proximally to involve the entire colon (pancolitis), no skip lesions as in Crohn's, red granular mucosa with superficial ulceration and pseudopolyps (islands of non-ulcerated swollen mucosa).
Micro: Acute and chronic inflammatory cells in lamina propria, inflamed areas are contiguous, crypt abscesses (neutrophils in colonic glands), cell dysplasia in those with long history.

I: **Bloods:** FBC (↓ Hb, ↑ WCC), ↑ ESR or CRP, ↓ albumin, crossmatch if severe blood loss, LFT.
Stool: Culture (for *Escherichia coli* 0157, *Campylobacter* and *Shigella*) and *Clostridium difficile* toxin as infectious colitis is a differential diagnosis.
AXR: To rule out toxic megacolon (see Toxic megacolon).
Flexible sigmoidoscopy or colonoscopy (and biopsy): Determines severity, histological confirmation, detection of dysplasia.
Barium enema: Mucosal ulceration with granular appearance and filling defects (pseudopolyps), featureless narrowed colon, loss of haustral pattern (leadpipe or hosepipe appearance) (see Fig. 30). Colonoscopy and barium enema may be dangerous in acute exacerbations (risk of perforation).
Radio-labelled white cell scan: Highlights areas of bowel inflammation.

M: **Markers of activity:** ↓ Hb, ↓ alb, ↑ ESR or CRP and diarrhoea frequency (< 4 per day is mild, 4–6 per day is moderate, > 6 per day is severe), bleeding, fever.
Acute exacerbation: Nil by mouth, IV rehydration, IV corticosteroids, parenteral feeding may be necessary, antibiotics and DVT prophylaxis. Monitor fluid balance and vital signs closely. Bowel resection if there is toxic megacolon as perforation has a mortality of 30%.
Mild attacks: Oral or rectal 5-ASA (e.g. sulphasalazine) or rectal steroids.
Moderate attacks: Oral steroids and oral 5-ASA.
Maintenance of remission: 5-ASA, consider other immunosuppressants (e.g. cyclosporin, azathioprine).
Advice: Patient education and support. Treatment of complications. Regular colonoscopic surveillance.
Surgical: Indicated for failure of medical treatment, presence of complications or prevention of colonic carcinoma. Proctocolectomy with ileostomy or an ileo-anal pouch formation provides good results.

CONDITIONS

C: **Gastrointestinal:** Haemorrhage, toxic megacolon, perforation, colonic carcinoma (in those with extensive disease for > 10 years), gallstones and PSC.
Extra-gastrointestinal manifestations (10–20%): Uveitis, renal calculi, arthropathy, sacroiliitis, ankylosing spondylitis, erythema nodosum, pyoderma gangrenosum, osteoporosis (from steroid treatment), amyloidosis.

P: A relapsing and remitting condition, with normal life expectancy.
Poor prognostic factors **(ABCDEF)**: **A**lbumin (< 30 g/L), **B**lood PR, **C**RP raised, **D**ilated loops of bowel, **E**ight or more bowel movements per day, **F**ever (> 38°C in first 24 h).

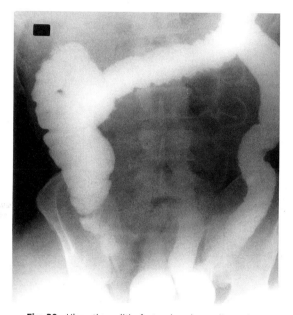

Fig. 30 Ulcerative colitis: featureless descending colon.

D: Involuntary urine loss following a rise in intra-abdominal pressure.

A: Developmental or damage to the bladder neck support.

A/R: Associated with vaginal prolapse in 50% of cases. Multiparity ↑ the risk of developing urinary stress incontinence.

E: Very common (25% of older women suffer from mild symptoms, 5–10% with severe symptoms). Uncommon in men.

H: Involuntary loss of urine associated with a sudden rise in intra-abdominal pressure (e.g. coughing, sneezing, lifting). A patient can be asked to keep a fluid diary: asking patient to record intake, times and volumes of urine passed and episodes of incontinence.

E: Urinary leakage on coughing, there may be an associated cystocoele on speculum examination.

P: Raised intra-abdominal pressure is not adequately transmitted to the proximal urethra, resulting in a disproportionate rise of bladder pressure over urethral pressure. Also, the descent of the urethra–vesical junction (from weakness in the pelvic floor muscles) results in a loss of normal sphincter closure. This is exacerbated during pregnancy, as progesterone promotes relaxation of the bladder and proximal urethral muscles.

I: **Urinalysis:** To exclude infection and glycosuria.
Imaging: MRI pelvis.
Urodynamic studies: To differentiate from other forms of urinary incontinence if the diagnosis is unclear.

M: **Conservative:** For mild symptoms, pelvic floor exercises are recommended to strengthen levator ani muscles. Intra-abdominal pressure is ↓ by weight reduction, avoiding excessive physical exertion and treating excessive coughing or sneezing.
Medical: *Hormone Replacement Therapy*: May be effective in postmenopausal women with urogenital atrophy.
Anticholinergic (e.g. imipramine): ↑ Urethral and bladder neck tone and relaxes detrusor muscles, thereby improving symptoms.
Surgical: *Retropubic bladder neck suspension*: Achieved by suturing the perivesical fascia to the pectineal ligament (Burch colposuspension) or suturing the periurethral fascia to the posterior surface of the symphysis pubis (Marshall–Marchetti–Krantz operation).
Sling operations: Insertion of synthetic material or natural tissue around the bladder and urethra, which are attached to the anterior rectus fascia supporting and partially compressing the urethra. It is indicated for patients with intrinsic sphincter damage or weakness.
Anterior colporrhaphy: Effective in patients with other prolapses as it also corrects these conditions.

C: **From surgery:** Obstructed voiding on micturition.

P: In mild cases, pelvic floor exercises will cure 40% and provide significant improvement in 80% long term. Retropubic bladder neck suspensions have an 80–90% long-term success rate whereas anterior colporrhaphy has only a 40% long-term success rate.

CONDITIONS

Urinary tract calculi

D: Crystal deposition within the urinary tract. Also known as nephrolithiasis.

A: Many cases are idiopathic. Others:
Metabolic: Hypercalciuria, hyperuricaemia, hypercystinuria, hyperoxaluria.
Infection: Hyperuricaemia.
Anatomic factors: Hypercystinuria, hyperoxaluria.
Drugs: Indinavir.

A/R: Risk factors include low fluid intake, structural urinary tract anomalies (e.g. horseshoe kidney, medullary sponge kidney).

E: Common. Prevalence is about 2–3% of the population per year. Male : female is 3 : 1. Lifetime risk is 10–15% in men, 5–10% in women. Age group affected is 20–50 years. Bladder stones are more common in developing countries, upper tract stones in industrialised countries.

H: Often asymptomatic.
Severe 'loin to groin' flank pain (renal pain, caliceal or ureteric colic), may be associated with nausea and vomiting when pain is severe.
Urinary urgency, frequency or retention.
Haematuria.

E: Loin or lower abdominal tenderness, without signs of peritonism. A leaking AAA is the most important differential diagnosis to consider in older men. Signs of systemic sepsis if there is obstruction and infection above a stone.

P: Calculi are formed by the supersaturation of urine by stone-forming compounds allowing crystallisation around a focus (e.g. infection, tumour, foreign bodies).
Main types of stones:
Calcium oxalate: Commonest type. Sharp projections often causing surrounding trauma. Also known as 'mulberry' stones.
Struvite (magnesium, ammonia, phosphate): Common. Smooth and dirty white in colour. Associated with urea-splitting bacteria, e.g. *Proteus*, *Pseudomonas*, *Klebsiella*. May form 'staghorn' stones within the kidneys.
Calcium phosphate.
Urate: Uncommon (5%). Hard, smooth, brown and faceted. Occurs in acidic urine.
Cystine: Uncommon (2%). White and translucent. Occurs in acidic urine.

I: **Blood:** FBC (raised WCC indicates possible infection), U&Es (to assess renal function) Ca^{2+}, urate, PO_4^{3-} (if raised warrants further investigation for causes).
Urine: Dipstick (if no haematuria, diagnosis is questionable), culture and sensitivity, 24-h urine collection (for calculi and to measure calculi-forming ion levels).
Radiology: KUB: 80% of stones are radio-opaque and will show up on a plain radiograph of the lower abdomen and pelvis.
IVU: Enables visualisation of kidneys and ureters. In the presence of a ureteric stone, can be a delayed dense nephrogram phase, with later films showing a dilated pelvicaliceal system and a standing column of contrast down to the site of the stone (see Fig. 31).
Ultrasound: Can also show ureteral dilation or hydronephrosis resulting from an obstructive uropathy; however, not sensitive for detecting smaller stones. Used in patients in whom IVU contrast is contraindicated.
Non-enhanced spiral CT: Also used to image stones but has higher radiation dose.
Isotope renography (e.g. with DTPA or DMSA)**:** Used in assessment of kidney function in complex stone disease.

M: **Acute presentation:** Analgesia, bed rest and fluid replacement (oral or IV). Urine collection to retrieve any calculi passed for analysis. Suitable for stones not causing obstruction; with the majority < 5 mm will pass this way. An obstructed infected kidney should be treated as an emergency with urgent relief of obstruction, e.g. by placement of a percutaneous nephrostomy under radiological guidance with antibiotic and other supportive measures.

Removal of calculi: Active intervention is indicated if the calculi obstructs or there is continuing pain or pyrexia.

Urethroscopy: Flexible or rigid urethroscope is passed into the bladder and up the ureter to visualise the stone. It can then be removed by a basket, grasper or broken up with laser, ultrasound or other methods. If the stone is impacted and cannot be removed, a JJ stent should be placed to ensure urine drainage.

Extracorporeal shock-wave lithotripsy: Non-invasive. An electromagnetic or piezoelectric shock wave is focused onto calculus to break it up into smaller fragments than can pass spontaneously. Suitable for stones < 2 cm as long as no obstruction to drainage.

Percutaneous nephrolithotomy: Performed for large complex stones, e.g. staghorn calculi. Following creation of a nephrostomy tract, a nephroscope is introduced and allows disintegration and removal of stones. A nephrostomy tube is left in situ for 1–2 days post op, with a nephrostogram performed to ensure stone removal and confirm normal ureteric drainage.

Open nephro-, pyelo- or ureterolithotomy: Less commonly performed, usually for complex stones.

Nephrectomy may be indicated in a nonfunctioning kidney.

Treatment of cause: Depends on the cause; e.g. parathyroidectomy, dietary calcium or oxalate restriction, allopurinol. Urine alkalinisation with oral potassium citrate is useful in dissolving urate and cystine stones.

Advice: Encourage high oral fluid intake.

C: **Of stones:** Infection, especially pyelonephritis, septicaemia, urinary retention.

Of ureteroscopy: Perforation, false passage.

Of lithotripsy: Pain, haematuria, Steinstrasse (ureteric obstruction caused by a column of stone fragments).

P: Generally good, but infection of renal calculi can potentially lead to irreversible renal scarring. Recurrence rate is about 50% within 5 years.

CONDITIONS

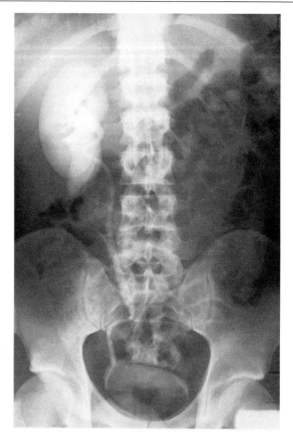

Fig. 31 IVU: right obstructed kidney with nephrogram and standing column.

D: Veins that have become prominantly elongated, dilated and tortuous; most commonly the superficial veins of the lower limbs. Thread veins, 'spider veins' or reticular veins refer to smaller superficial venous telangiectasias and varicosities.

A: **Primary:** Due to genetic or developmental weakness in the vein wall resulting in ↓ elasticity, dilation over time and valvular incompetence.
Secondary: *Venous outflow obstruction*: Pregnancy, pelvic malignancy, ovarian cysts, ascites, lymphadenopathy, retroperitoneal fibrosis.
Valve damage: After DVT.
High flow: Arteriovenous fistula.

A/R: Age, female, family history, race (↑ Caucasians), obesity.

E: Common, ↑ with age, prevalence: 10–15% adult men, 20–25% adult women.

H: Patient may complain about cosmetic appearance or experience symptoms such as aching in the legs, worse towards the end of the day or after standing for long periods; swelling, itching, or complications such as bleeding, infection or ulceration.

E: **Inspection:** Inspect with the patient standing.
Palpation: Fascial defects along the dilated veins, the sites of incompetent perforators, may be palpated. A cough impulse may be felt over the SFJ. The tap test refers to an impulse felt distally along the vein after tapping over the SFJ (normally not present due to competent valves). Presence of foot pulses should be documented. Palpation of a thrill or auscultation of a bruit suggests an AV fistula.
Trendelenburg test: Can localise sites of valvular incompetence. With the patient supine, the leg is elevated and the veins emptied, a hand/tourniquet is used to compress the SFJ, the leg is placed in the dependent position and filling of the veins observed before or after the tourniquet/hand is released. Hand-held Doppler can sensitively demonstrate SFJ incompetence.
Rectal or pelvic examination: May be performed if secondary causes are suspected.
Signs of venous insufficiency: Varicose eczema, hemosiderin staining, atrophie blanche, lipodermatosclerosis, oedema, ulceration.

P: Theories on pathogenesis of varicose veins include primary valvular incompetence and the development of weakness of the vein wall due to abnormalities of collagen and elastin with fibrosis of the tunica media in advanced stages. Other factors including venous hypertension and hormonal changes are also implicated.

I: **Duplex ultrasound:** Locates sites of incompetence or reflux. Also to exclude DVT (important if surgery contemplated).

M: **Conservative:** Advice on exercise (improves the calf muscle pump) and elevation of the legs at rest. Class II support stockings can be used to aid venous return.
Venous telangiectasia and reticular veins: Microinjection or laser sclerotherapy.
Surgical: The veins are marked with the patient in the standing postion prior to operation. SFJ ligation, stripping of the long saphenous vein to the knee and avulsion of varicosities via small stab incisions is performed. The short saphenous vein is not stripped, just ligated to avoid potential damage to the sural nerve. Post-op, the legs are bandaged and early mobilisation encouraged. Subfascial endoscopic perforator surgery is a more recent development involving ligation of incompetent perforating veins using an endoscopic technique.

C: Venous pigmentation, eczema, lipodermatosclerosis, superficial thrombophlebitis, venous ulceraton.
Of treatment: *Sclerotherapy*: Skin staining, local scarring. *Surgery*: Haemorrhage, infection, recurrence (5–30%), paraesthesia (6%), peroneal nerve injury (0.1%).

P: In general, slowly progressive. Recurrence rates post surgery can be up to 40%.

I: **Elective:** Contraception (should be considered irreversible).
Rarely, it can be used to treat recurrent epididymitis (reduces risk by 60%).

A: The vas deferens (ductus deferens) is a duct delivering spermatozoa produced in the testes, from the tail of the epididymis to the ejaculatory ducts. It is 45 cm long and traverses the scrotum and inguinal canal. It crosses the external iliac artery, entering the pelvis below the peritoneum covering the lateral wall. At the ischial tuberosity, it turns medially, crosses in front of the ureter to the base of the bladder where it joins the ipsilateral seminal vesicle to form the ejaculatory duct that travels through the prostate gland to open into the prostatic urethra. The artery to the vas is from the internal iliac artery and it may be encapsulated by varicosities, i.e. varicocele in the scrotum.

I: Performed under local anaesthesia.
Pre-op: Patient and partner should be counselled. It should be stressed to the patient that this procedure should be considered irreversible. Medical history is reviewed and certain medication stopped, e.g. aspirin 1 week pre-op.
Skin should be shaved and cleaned with antiseptic.
Post-op: Scrotal support is worn for up to 1 week. Patient should be warned to continue using pre-op contraceptive methods for ~ 12 weeks and two separate semen samples should confirm azoospermia.

P: The two techniques are scalpel and no-scalpel:
Scalpel: The vas deferens is held between thumb and two fingers, and local anaesthetic is infiltrated, usually at the junction of the middle and upper ⅓ of the scrotum bilaterally. A small vertical incision is made over the vas on the scrotal surface. Surrounding tissue is bluntly dissected away, the vas deferens drawn out of the incision and a clip is used to grasp the midportion. The vas is ligated and a length excised (usually ~ 1–2 cm). Cauterisation to the cut ends, folding back the vas or fascial interposition are used to prevent recanalisation. Skin closure is achieved with simple interrupted sutures. This is repeated on the other side.
No-scalpel: Vas deferens is palpated under the skin and clamped with a ring forceps. Skin is pierced with dissecting forceps and used to create an opening. Vas is drawn out and treated as with the scalpel technique.
The excised segment of vas should be sent for histological confirmation.

C: **Short-term:** Infection, bruising, bleeding/haematoma, sperm granuloma, epididymitis.
Long-term: < 1% failure rate (i.e. conception) due to recanalisation, surgical error, anatomical variants or failure of contraception prior to confirmation of azoospermia. Scrotal pain is uncommon.

PROCEDURES

I: Rupture of the transverse ligament.
Atlanto-axial instability (distance between posterior segment of anterior arch of C1 to anterior segment of odontoid process of C2 is > 5 mm on lateral cervical spine X-ray).

A: **Atlas:** The 1st cervical vertebra (the atlas) is a ring of bone with anterior and posterior arches, and a lateral mass on either side with articular surfaces above and below to form the atlanto-occipital and atlanto-axial joints. The atlas has no vertebral body or spinous process.
Axis: The odontoid process arises from the body of the 2nd cervical vertebra (the axis), effectively being the vertebral body of the atlas that has fused with the axis.
Ligaments: Anterior and posterior longitudinal ligaments run down the anterior and posterior surface of the vertebral bodies: the ligamenta flava connect the vertebral laminae, and in the cervical spine the ligamentum nuchae connects the spinous processes and runs from the 7th cervical vertebra to the external occipital protuberance.
Atlanto-axial joint: Within the atlanto-axial joint, the transverse part of the cruciate ligament is attached bilaterally to the inner surface of the lateral mass, binding the odontoid process to the anterior arch of the atlas preventing anterior subluxation of the atlas on the axis.

I: **Pre-op:** General anaesthetic assessment. Lateral view of cervical spine (flexion and extension) allows diagnosis of atlanto-axial instability.
Post-op: DVT prophylaxis. A brace or hard collar is worn for 8–12 weeks and a repeat radiograph is performed after removal.

P: **Position:** The patient is positioned prone with the neck in a slightly flexed position for posterior cervical exposure. Radiographs of the spine are taken to confirm its position.
Incision and exposure: A midline incision and dissection is performed down to the spinous process and laminae of the axis and the posterior tubercle of the atlas. These are dissected free from all soft tissue. The posterior arch of the atlas is exposed subperiosteally with dissection carefully carried out on the lower border of the atlas.
Fusion and bone graft: The anterior surface of the posterior arch is carefully dissected free from the periosteum and a channel is made from inferior to superior. An 18-gauge stainless steel wire is bent into a U-shape and the loop is passed through the channel from inferior to superior. A unicortical piece of bone is extracted from the posterior iliac crest and shaped to fit between the tubercle of the atlas and the spinous process of the axis. The posterior surface of the atlas and axis is decorticated and the bone graft is fitted over the posterior elements. The loop of wire is passed over the graft and hooped around the spinous process of the axis. The ends of the wire are then pulled around either sides of the bone graft and twisted together securing the graft.
Closure: The wound is closed and a brace/hard collar is used post-op for 8–12 weeks.

C: Infection, damage to vertebral arteries.

P: Successful fusion rate of 90–100%. There is some loss of cervical rotation.

D: Rotation of a loop of bowel around the axis of its mesentery that resuls in bowel obstruction and potential ischaemia. The areas usually affected in adults are the sigmoid colon (65%) and caecum (30%). In neonates (volvulus neonatorum), midgut volvulus is more common.

A: Anatomical factors, such as a long mesentery, sometimes due to adhesions or tumour. Volvulus neonatorum is due to malrotation of the embryonic gut during development.

A/R: **Adults:** Long sigmoid colon and mesentery, mobile caecum, chronic constipation and debility, very high residue diet, tumour, adhesions, Chagas' disease of the colon and parasitic infections.
Neonatal: Associated with malrotation and Ladd's bands (peritoneal bands from the caecum to the posterior abdominal wall that cross over the duodenum).

E: **Adult:** Causes $\sim$5% of LBO, more common in the elderly and in Africa and Asia.
Neonatal: Rare, incidence of 5.7/100 000, with a male predominance.

P: Rotation of the segment of bowel results in partial or complete closed loop obstruction. With a 360° twist, the veins to the bowel are compressed and occluded leading to circulatory impairment and if not relieved, gangrene and perforation. In neonatal volvulus, malrotation causes the duodenojejunal junction to lie on the right of the midline and the caecum in the upper abdomen, with resulting narrow midgut mesenteric base and predisposing to volvulus.

H: Severe colicky abdominal pain and swelling, absolute constipation, and later, vomiting. There may be a history of transient attacks in which spontaneous reduction of the volvulus has occurred. Neonatal volvulus presents at $\sim$3months with distress due to pain and bile-stained vomiting.

E: Signs of bowel obstruction with abdominal distension and tenderness.
Absent or frequent loud tinkling bowel sounds.
Fever, tachycardia, signs of dehydration.

I: **Imaging: AXR:** Shows a single greatly dilated loop of bowel, which in large bowel volvulus may have a 'coffee bean' shape. In caecal volvulus, the concavity of the coffee bean points to the right lower quadrant and in sigmoid, to the left. May be associated with proximally dilated loops of bowel and distal collapse.
Erect CXR: If perforation is suspected.
Water-soluble contrast enema: Demonstrates the site of obstruction; in sigmoid volvulus, there is a 'bird's beak' or 'ace of spades' deformity with spiral narrowing of the distal bowel at the site.
CT scan: Can identify rotation and torsion of mesentery and bowel as well as signs suggestive of infarction.

M: **Resuscitation:** Nil by mouth, IV fluid, NG tube if vomiting.
Conservative: IV broad-spectrum antibiotics (e.g. cephalosporin and metronidazole) if signs of sepsis. Sigmoid volvulus may be managed by endoscopic placement of a flatus tube for decompression. Recurrent cases should be treated by elective sigmoid colectomy.
Surgical: Urgent laparotomy and untwisting of the bowel. Any gangrenous or ischaemic bowel is resected, with either a primary anastomosis and/or stoma formation. In the case of caecal volvulus, right hemicolectomy, caecopexy (fixation by suturing to the posterior peritoneum) or caecostomy is performed.
Neonatal: At laparotomy, volvulus is corrected by rotating anticlockwise with division of associated bands. If viable, the small bowel is placed on the

right and the caecum and colon to the left, widening the mesenteric base, performing appendicectomy, as it now lies on the left. If a region of bowel is frankly ischaemic, excision is performed. To avoid extensive resection, the bowel may be returned and a second-look laparotomy performed in 24–48 h.

C: Bowel obstruction, ischaemia and gangrene, toxaemia, bowel perforation, peritonitis, short gut syndrome if extensive small bowel resection.

P: Overall mortality of 10–35%. >40% mortality in gangrenous intestinal volvulus.

I: Single primary breast tumour, generally < 4 cm in diameter that can be excised with clear resection margins > 5 mm (ideally 1 cm), and produce satisfactory cosmetic results, and for the patient to be suitable for post-op radiotherapy and follow-up.

A: The mammary gland consists of 15–20 lobes radiating outwards from the nipple. Each lobe is separated from the other by fibrous septa and from the underlying muscle by the retromammary space. The base of the breast covers the 2nd to the 6th rib and the lateral sternal margin to the mid-axillary line. The axillary tail (of Spence) runs upwards and laterally into the deep fascia at the lower border of pectoralis major muscle coming into close relation with the axillary vessels.

Vascular: The arterial supply and corresponding venous drainage are from the perforating arteries of the internal thoracic, intercostal and axillary arteries.

Lymphatics: Lymphatics of the lateral half drains into the anterior axillary and pectoral nodes while the medial half drains into the nodes along the internal thoracic artery. There is lymphatic drainage into the lymph vessels of the opposite breast as well as drainage posteriorly along the posterior intercostals artery into the posterior intercostal nodes.

I: **Pre-op:** Patients will have had triple assessment of clinical examination, imaging (mammogram or ultrasound) and cytogical analysis of FNA or trucut biopsy. With smaller, impalpable lesion, wire localisation under imaging may be required on the morning of the operation. FBC, U&Es, G&S and clotting should be performed. CXR and ECG in older individuals. General anaesthetic assessment.

Post-op: DVT prophylaxis. Needle aspiration of tissue fluid collections is commonly required.

P: **Access:** An elliptical incision is made directly over the breast mass following the line of skin tension. There is usually no excision of skin except if needed to achieve an adequate tumour-free margin.

Excision: Dissection is performed to remove a block of breast tissue containing the lesion with an ellipse of normal tissue surrounding it, allowing for adequate margins. The removed block of tissue should be marked with sutures to allow orientation on histological analysis. Meticulous haemostasis in the remaining cavity is achieved with any exposed muscle at the base of the cavity being covered with breast tissue.

Closure: Sutures placed to close the dead space. The wound is closed in two layers with absorbable sutures: the dermis with buried interrupted sutures and the skin with continuous subcuticular sutures.

Axillary node sampling and clearance: Axillary node dissection is now carried out usually through a separate incision behind the lateral border of pectoralis major. The levels of axillary clearance are defined in relation to pectoralis minor, level 1 nodes up to the muscle, level II nodes behind it and level III nodes beyond pectoralis minor up to subclavius. Positive nodes in a level I clearance require radiotherapy while level III clearance obviates need for further axillary treatment. In all levels the axillary vein is distinguished, with careful identification of the long thoracic nerve of Bell (to serratus anterior) and the thoracodorsal nerve and vessels (supply latissimus dorsi). The intercostobrachial nerve runs laterally through the axilla and may need to be sacrificed.

C: Wound infection, haemorrhage, poor skin healing and cosmetic result. Of axillary surgery: frozen shoulder, axilla pain, arm lymphoedema, damage to the long thoracic nerve can result in a winged scapula.